EMPOWERING

PRACTICE IN

SOCIAL CARE

EMPOWERING

PRACTICE IN

SOCIAL CARE

Suzy Braye and
Michael Preston-Shoot

Open University Press
Buckingham • Philadelphia

Open University Press
Celtic Court
22 Ballmoor
Buckingham
MK18 1XW

and
1900 Frost Road, Suite 101
Bristol, PA 19007, USA

First Published 1995

A catalogue record for this book is available from the British Library

ISBN   0 335 19245 9 (pb)   0 335 19246 7 (hb)

Library of Congress Cataloging-in-Publication Data
Braye, Suzy, 1950–
    Empowering practice in social care / Suzy Braye and Michael
Preston-Shoot.
        p. cm.
    Includes bibliographical references and index.
    ISBN 0–335–19246–7. — ISBN 0–335–19245–9 (pbk.)
        1. Social service—Great Britain.   2. Human services—Great
Britain.   3. Community organization—Great Britain.
    4. Neighborhood—Great Britain.   I. Preston-Shoot, Michael.
    II. Title.
    HV245.B7625   1995
    361.94—dc20   94–28838
                                                                    CIP

Typeset by Graphicraft Typesetters Ltd., Hong Kong
Printed in Great Britain by Biddles Ltd., Guildford and King's Lynn

Contents

Acknowledgements

Learning and writing about empowering practice has been, and will continue to be, both challenging and necessary to us in both professional and personal capacities. From the perspective of being white professionals, one of us a woman, one a man, we must acknowledge how others have contributed to our learning from both similar and different perspectives. In particular, Ann Plumb, Andrew Hughes, Jane Kenny and Mary Varley have been generous in partnerships we have much appreciated and valued. Members of the Staff Development Team of Stockport Social Services Department provided an empowering environment for developing ideas and understanding. We are grateful to Jean Fullwood for unravelling the mysteries of National Vocational Qualifications, and to Dianne Moss and Trish Carabine for typing parts of this book. Jo Campling again gave us her confidence and encouraged ours.

Two chapters in the book develop substantially thinking which we have previously published elsewhere. We are grateful to the editors and publishers for permission to quote from our articles in the *Journal of Social Work Practice*, published by Carfax, PO Box 25, Abingdon, Oxon, and the *Journal of Social Welfare and Family Law*, published by Routledge (Braye and Preston-Shoot 1993b, 1994).

We must also thank those who provided practical and moral support: Ann and Vic, Linda and Vic, Jill and Michael, Ali and David, Margaret and Bill, and Eileen and John.

Our special thanks are due to Hannah and Sebastian for saving the best fun until we had finished the book.

Suzy Braye and Michael Preston-Shoot

Abbreviations

AHRA	Access to Health Records Act 1990
APFA	Access to Personal Files Act 1987
BASW	British Association of Social Workers
CA	Children Act 1989
CCETSW	Central Council for Education and Training in Social Work
CSDPA	Chronically Sick and Disabled Persons Act 1970
DHA	District health authority
DHSS	Department of Health and Social Security
DoH	Department of Health
DPA(SCR)	Disabled Persons (Services, Consultation and Representation) Act 1986
FHSA	Family health services authority
HSPHA	Health Services and Public Health Act 1968
LBTC	London Borough Training Consortium
MHA	Mental Health Act 1983
MISG	Mental Illness Special Grant
NAA	National Assistance Act 1948
NAREA	National Association of Race Equality Advisers
NCC	National Consumer Council
NCVQ	National Council for Vocational Qualifications
NCVS	Nottingham Council for Voluntary Service
NHSA	National Health Service Act 1977
NHSCCA	NHS and Community Care Act 1990
NHSTD	National Health Service Training Directorate
NISW/NEC	National Institute for Social Work/National Extension College
NUPE	National Union of Public Employees
NVQ	National Vocational Qualifications

OSDC	Organisation and Social Development Consultants
REU	Race Equality Unit
RRA	Race Relations Act 1976
SDA	Sex Discrimination Act 1975
SOA	Sexual Offences Act 1956
SSD	Social services department
SSI	Social Services Inspectorate
UPIAS	Union of the Physically Impaired Against Segregation

Cases

R. v. *Avon County Council, Ex parte Mark Hazell.*
R. v. *Secretary of State for Education and Science, Ex parte E* [1991] *The Guardian,* 10 May.

Introduction

Developments in community care ushered in by the NHS and Community Care Act 1990 and its associated guidance have brought radical changes to the relationship between local authorities and independent agencies, and between practitioners, service users and their carers. They have required changes in the functions of social services departments and, therefore, also necessitated the development of different staff job roles. While government policy documents present them as unproblematic and straightforward, negotiating these developments and changes is far from being a simple process.

Policy creates one set of demands on practitioners and managers by posing at a conceptual level a range of conflicting imperatives which give rise at a practical level to dilemmas and tensions. Community care is a broad concept which masks differing ideologies and meanings. Need and choice are juxtaposed with economy and efficiency in the use of resources. Power to determine provision remains with professionals rather than users, potentially undermining the emphasis on user self-determination. Assumptions about 'family' and 'community' reflect stereotypical understandings about roles and relationships, ignoring dimensions of gender, race and class which impact upon people's lives. Effective service provision depends on efficient mechanisms for collaboration between professionals and their agencies, yet structures and funding emphasize separate and often diverging systems of responsibility and accountability. The rhetoric may be one of partnership, choice and a seamless service. The contradictions demonstrate the competing and complex influences which underpin policy, reflecting a confusion of terms and intentions, leaving tensions unresolved, and acting as disincentives to empowering practice.

Further demands on practitioners derive from the emergence of a strong value base in social care, concerned with how power and authority are used in caring professions, and how practice can challenge inequality and oppression. Yet available legislation and policy is partial in its support for anti-discriminatory practice and silent in relation to anti-oppressive practice. Services continue to cater for dominant social groups and to be primarily functionalist, using a 'fix it' model of cure or care for individual symptoms and problems, rather than enabling service users to tackle the structures which oppress them and limit their opportunities. Moreover, the value base itself is under attack.

Upon what help can staff draw? Policy guidance largely focuses on management and organizational issues, with little attention to the complexity of either the basic tasks undertaken by practitioners with users or the dilemmas which policy and legislation bequeath to practitioners. Where roles and skills are expounded they are those of purchasers rather than providers of care, perpetuating longstanding assumptions that provider skills are those of everyday common sense. Similarly, where guidance mentions underpinning values of the service, it places these in the guardianship of purchasers who are seen as responsible for quality assurance by imposing strict standards upon providers and inspecting their performance. This is a simplistic and partial view. Service providers appear as relatively powerless, a perception which does little justice to the complexity of the care provision task. Moreover, it is complacent given known abuses in residential and domiciliary care, and legal judgements which have found local authorities failing to meet their statutory obligations. While attention is given to the development of structures and mechanisms to assist inter-agency collaboration, little help is given to practitioners in their task of interdisciplinary cooperation at a day-to-day level. These issues are debilitating for staff and users alike, and threaten to undermine the possibilities presented by the policy changes, for in such situations practitioners are less likely to be user-focused and more inclined to practise defensively or in accordance with agency instructions.

Standards of qualifying competence have been developed for social care workers. While these recognize the interrelatedness of knowledge, attitudes and skills as components of competence, and the influence of the organizational context, they are presented as if unproblematic and mutually consistent and supportive. Staff are left to appreciate and negotiate the sometimes contradictory requirements for practice competence. Existing literature for social care purchasers and providers does not address the subject in the complexity or comprehensiveness it requires: to enable practitioners to understand and negotiate the changes introduced by government policy; to translate core values into empowering skills; to maintain a questioning, analytical stance on social care; and to connect, in a practical and principled manner, individual and social change.

This book will bring together the major tensions, dilemmas and themes within the provision of social care, and will juxtapose these with the values, knowledge and skills which will guide practitioners through these complex issues as they present in the work experience. It will address the job roles and functions of staff providing social care, and enable a critical understanding of the complexities, tensions and dilemmas of the task, and of the assumptions and ideologies which underpin the development of community care.

It will encourage workers to negotiate the power dynamics of their relationship with users, to develop skills in working within the ethos of empowerment and partnership. It will assist workers with the interprofessional and inter-agency collaboration that is essential for the effective provision of care, and will identify the elements of a competent context for practice.

Some reference is necessary to the terminology used in this book. There is an ongoing debate on the respective merits of 'client', 'service user' and 'consumer'. While none of these terms fully reflects the relationship between those who provide and receive social care, this book will employ the term 'service user'. This appears to enjoy more widespread acceptance although, arguably, it inaccurately conveys the nature of the relationship with practitioners when compulsion is involved.

The book adopts the term 'black' to describe someone whose skin colour exposes him or her to racism, irrespective of other ethnic and cultural factors. Some communities are not so visible but none the less experience discrimination and inequality as a result of their ethnicity, national origin, language, culture or religion. The book uses the terms 'disabled people' and 'people with learning disabilities' since these terms are preferred by people themselves. 'Emotional distress' or 'mental health problems' are terms used in preference to psychiatric terminology or the label 'mental illness' to describe the experiences of people who encounter distress of a degree that brings them into contact with psychiatric services. The term 'survivor' is used to validate the strength of people who are resolving their distress or surviving the psychiatric system. 'Older people' or 'old people' is preferred to any term, such as 'the elderly', which attempts to categorize people in one homogeneous group. Terminologies must reflect a respect for diversity, an understanding of the political function of language and the expressed preferences of people they attempt to represent and describe.

The book takes it as axiomatic that inequality and oppression in the form of racism, sexism, ageism, disablism, mentalism and heterosexism exist at individual and structural levels; that is, that they occur between people, and are expressed through organizational policy and practice and through society's institutions. Accordingly, key themes will permeate the book: anti-oppressive practice, individual and structural change, partnership, empowerment and power. These themes will be elaborated and applied to the interactions between practitioners and users.

Each chapter will contain several exercises which readers are recommended to consider before progressing further through the book. They may be used by individual readers, or as training exercises for groups. They are designed to enable readers to identify and develop the values, knowledge and skills which comprise the social care task, to develop their understanding of the practice dilemmas in action, to tackle the decision-making and choices inherent in specific situations and to define the requirements of good practice.

The book contains three sections. The first, which follows now, sets the scene by appraising the overarching policy mandates and underpinning values, together with the training and organizational context for practice development.

Part I Overarching mandates

and values

The three chapters in this section each take a key element of social care practice and subject it to critical scrutiny. Chapter 1 focuses on the legislative and policy context, providing an analysis of its core components, and revealing that this mandate for social care is neither straightforward nor unproblematic.

Chapter 2 focuses on the different values upon which welfare professionals may draw, identifying tensions between values which maintain a status quo in social relations and those which express a commitment to social change, needs-led services and anti-oppressive practice. Once again, what characterizes this analysis are the choices and dilemmas faced by practitioners attempting to integrate values arising from differing moral perspectives. The resulting complexity has implications, to which this chapter draws attention, for the ways in which practitioners and managers conceptualize models for understanding the social care task, the organizational context, and their personal experience.

The theme of Chapter 3 is the importance of training and staff development for service providers as well as purchasers, if the dilemmas in practice resulting from the confused policy and values mandates are to inspire rather than defeat practitioners and managers in their objective of empowering practice in social care. Once again, a critical analysis is undertaken of the trends in, and content of, training, coupled with an articulation of how organizations can promote competent practice, with particular reference to agency practice and staff development.

Social care is a complex and challenging endeavour. The critique provided in this section illustrates the assumptions and confusions contained in legislation and policy guidance, the challenge if the potential of the value base is to be realized, and the ways in which organizations may succeed or fail to provide an empowering context for social care. It provides the foundation for critical reflective practice which reaches for an empowering relationship between service providers and service users.

1 Social care:

the policy context

The NHS and Community Care Act 1990 and associated volumes of guidance lay the foundation for the provision of care, services and resources to people who have needs arising from ill-health, ageing or disability. They provide the legal and policy context for social care provision, which is seen, along with health care, as a key component of good quality community care.

Community care means 'providing the services and support which people who are affected by problems of ageing, mental illness, mental handicap or physical disability need to be able to live as independently as possible in their own homes or in homely settings in the community' (DoH 1989a). In later policy documents the term mental handicap is replaced by learning disability.

Within the umbrella term community care, health care services are the responsibility of health authorities and social care services are the responsibility of local authority social services departments. Definitions of social care are scarce in government documentation. The term appears to encompass any non-medical provision given by health and welfare workers, ranging from domiciliary support to people in their own homes, respite care and day care for those with intensive care needs, through sheltered housing, group homes and hostels, to residential care, nursing homes and long-stay hospital care (DoH 1989a). The emphasis is on support for 'mobility, personal care, domestic tasks, financial affairs, accommodation, leisure and employment which [people] cannot arrange for themselves' (DoH 1989a). The key components of the system are services that:

- respond flexibly and sensitively to the needs of individuals and their carers;
- allow a wide range of options for consumers;
- intervene no more than necessary to foster independence;
- concentrate on those with greatest needs.

Social care has long been associated with social work. The Barclay enquiry (1982) into the roles and tasks of social workers identified *social care planning* as a key component, differentiated from the *counselling* role. Payne (1986) makes a similar distinction, equating social care with indirect social work, which focuses not just on individuals' behaviour, feelings and skills, but enables resources to be used more effectively in the provision of social services. This activity can either be focused on a service user's individual support network or take a wider social action perspective concerned with promoting social justice. This wide remit is echoed by an analysis of the aims and objectives of social care (Social Care Association 1988). These refer both to promoting health and welfare, and to minimizing the effects of social inequalities and oppression. The social care described in government guidance is very much the former, but no longer resides purely in the domain of social work, and the organizational context is markedly different.

Social services departments are responsible for ensuring that people who need social care services receive them. Service providers from the voluntary and independent sectors, as well as informal caring networks, are intended to play a major role in this provision. The local authority's *enabling* and coordinating role represents a shift from its traditional position as the major *provider* of services, and is at the heart of a number of mechanisms designed to ensure the achievement of key objectives (DoH 1989a):

- promoting the development of domiciliary, day and respite services to enable people to live in their own homes wherever feasible and sensible;
- ensuring that service providers make practical support for carers a high priority;
- making proper assessment of need and good case management the cornerstone of high quality care, with packages of care designed in line with individual needs and preferences;
- promoting the development of a flourishing independent sector alongside good quality public services;
- clarifying the responsibility of agencies and so making it easier to hold them accountable for their performance;
- securing better value for taxpayers' money by introducing a new funding structure for social care.

The local authority's role includes several key responsibilities. The local authority must:

- assess the need for social care services of people in its area;
- plan for the provision of services to meet those needs, establishing objectives and priorities;
- design packages of care, taking account of individuals' preferences;
- secure the delivery of appropriate services, either by direct provision or by purchasing services from others;
- assess service users' ability to contribute to the cost of those services;
- monitor the quality and cost-effectiveness of services;
- establish procedures for comment and complaint from service users.

Individuals requiring assistance which they are unable to arrange for themselves, whether that be domestic help or residential care, must undergo assessment by the local authority. Funding for this, additional to the local authority's core budget, derives from central government finance, ring-fenced until 1996, reflecting the care element of social security payments which would otherwise have been made to individuals entering private residential care under the previous funding system. From 1993 this finance was devolved to local authorities with the initial proviso that 85 per cent was to be spent in the independent sector, thus hastening the swing away from public provision. Additional 'start up' funding was also made available on a non-recurring basis. For service users with severe disabilities, local authorities must meet a proportion of the cost of the care package, with possible application to a new independent living fund for top up. The expectation is that packages costing over £500 (1993 costs) will trigger residential care.

This broad outline of some of the definitions and core components of the policy requires amplification and analysis. Interpretations vary: what is seen as a mixed economy of welfare controlled by people who use services may also be construed as a means of controlling expenditure on public provision. Such mixed perspectives derive partly from the diverse historical factors which influence the policy context.

Historical influences

The historical influences upon community care policy are complex, reflecting diverse and sometimes competing perspectives. By isolating the threads we can facilitate understanding of how they are woven together.

Much of the original impetus derived from debates on the appropriateness of institutional forms of care for people with mental health problems or learning difficulty (Levick 1992). Though the value of non-institutional life and care in the community had been articulated as a policy objective since the 1930s, it was not until the 1960s that momentum gathered (Baldwin and Parker 1990). A number of factors contributed to the widespread belief that non-institutional care was appropriate and achievable at this time and that investment in community facilities was necessary. The dehumanizing effects of institutional care were being recognized. Public scandals about the conditions and treatment of patients in large institutions contributed to this awareness, and to a politicized view of hospital care for people in emotional distress as an agency for worsening or even manufacturing pathology. In this respect the impetus for community care may be seen as a response to the political and professional guilt evoked by life within institutions (Ramon 1991a).

Developments in the manufacture of psychotropic drugs made it apparently possible to control the more overt symptoms of mental disorder, making physical restraint and isolation less necessary. As in other branches of medicine, success in acute treatment brought with it a changing emphasis to the more longstanding care implications of mental ill-health. It was recognized that patients deteriorated as much owing to preventable social factors, such as failure to provide after-care facilities, as to psychiatric disease processes. Increasing awareness of, and importance attached to, social factors in the aetiology and course of mental illness, together with evidence of widespread identifiable distress in the broad population, influenced the development of a new psychiatric ideology, which arguably (Prior 1993) was even more influential on the community care movement. In this analysis, if sanity and insanity are not clearly distinct categories with identifiable patterns of causation and treatment, asylums are no longer required to mark the boundary between them.

Other factors have exerted influence from different directions. Normalization values have had a major impact upon professional thinking, and thus upon policy development. The belief that disabled people have a right to experiences that are valued in society has had major implications for the living situations that are deemed acceptable, with inevitable support for non-institutional care. Advocacy and self-advocacy from users of services, in both the learning disability and mental health fields, have made similar contributions and led to growing recognition of demands for user participation in service development and delivery. Both of these factors will be explored further in Chapter 2.

Against this backdrop, policy developments were gradually gathering momentum. Between 1962, when the Hospital Plan for England and Wales promised the closure of psychiatric hospitals and their replacement by district general hospital units, hostels and day facilities, and 1975, government reports and White Papers were unanimous in setting targets to accelerate the shift from hospital to community care (DHSS 1971a, b, 1972, 1975). This period was characterized by consensus about the direction of policy and slow but consistent expansion of state welfare services (Langan 1990), making alternatives to hospital care possible and ensuring a gradual decline of the population in institutional care. The community care remit expanded to include other groups requiring long-term support without medical care, and the policy focus expanded to include the prevention of entry to institutional care as well as rehabilitation from it (Baldwin and Parker 1990).

Langan (1990) then identifies a second phase, one of retrenchment and stagnation, from the late 1970s to mid-1980s. Resource provision had already clearly lagged behind the planning vision. People discharged from hospitals were often being cared for by relatives with little state support, or were living alone in isolated and uncaring environments. Large numbers of people were remaining in hospitals who could be discharged if community facilities were available (DHSS 1981), but it was not until the Care in the Community Circular (DHSS 1983) that mechanisms for the necessary transfer of funding from health authorities to local authorities and voluntary bodies were devised. By now, however, the impact of spending cuts was being felt. During the period 1982–6 beds in psychiatric hospitals fell by 10,000, while day care provision increased by 543 places and residential care by 399 (Langan 1990). Increasing reliance was placed on informal networks of care, notably those provided by women, and on an expanding role for voluntary agencies as providers of services.

The apparent approving consensus about community care was increasingly tested, both by evidence of how it was operating in practice and by advocacy from groups such as the National Schizophrenia Fellowship, the Richmond Fellowship and, more recently, SANE (Schizophrenia a National Emergency) drawing attention to the distress caused by inadequately resourced 'rehabilitation' schemes.

The House of Commons Select Committee on Social Services, reporting on community care (1985), emphasized the need for expenditure, complained that government had provided little lead to clarify the services which local authorities should provide and warned against community care developing too quickly or on the cheap. The Audit Commission (1985), operating with the remit of identifying economy, efficiency and effectiveness in local authority services, noted that admission to residential care was sometimes made unnecessarily or prematurely through lack of spending on community care services. It also reported serious concerns about the slow progress of community care and poor value for money in this sector of public policy (Audit Commission 1986). It concluded that community care was not working for two reasons:

1 Funding arrangements were inadequate. First, there was 'a perverse financial incentive' in favour of residential care, which had resulted in an explosion of the numbers of people supported in private residential care on the basis of their financial eligibility rather than their need for such care. Second, the transfer since 1983 of funding from health to local authorities had serious shortcomings.
2 The shared responsibilities of health and social services were not working. There was organizational fragmentation and confusion at national, regional and local levels, compounded by complex local networks where boundaries were not conterminous. Differing organizational styles resulted in poor coordination and lack of trust, which led to patchy and inconsistent service development.

The Audit Commission's reports led directly to the establishment of a committee to review how public funds were used to support community care policy and to advise on options for improvement. The committee's report (Griffiths 1988) laid down the key foundation stones which are now reflected in official policy guidance. It paved the way for the change of role for local authorities, recommending they act 'as designers, organisers and purchasers of non-health care services, and not be primarily direct providers, making maximum possible use of voluntary and private sector bodies to widen consumer choice, stimulate innovation and encourage efficiency'. The White Paper (DoH 1989a) endorsed Griffiths's recommendations, which also underpin the subsequent legislation and policy guidance. This heralds the third phase in the historical development of community care, one of 'austerity and privatization' (Langan 1990), introducing a clearly demarcated two-tier system where those who can pay can choose, while those who need financial assistance must establish need.

The divergent themes in the historical development of thinking on community care are reflected in the confusions and ambiguities in core components of the policy. Differing influences have led to the term 'community care' having several different meanings, including where people live, what services they receive and who looks after them. Originally used to describe care outside large institutions, it is now commonly used to denote care in people's own homes, and other settings as close to ordinary living as possible. Besides describing a way of delivering services by professionals in non-hospital settings, it has also come to mean the involvement of members of the community in care-giving (Bulmer 1987), care by the community and care in the community (Bayley 1973). Its aims are ambitious and expansive, from rehabilitation of those who have been in institutional care to prevention for those at risk of entering it. It is framed both as enabling people to achieve maximum autonomy and independence through exercising choice, and as ensuring cost-effectiveness and value for money in spending from the public purse. The breadth of its definitions and meanings has ensured continued support from different quarters, used by the left as a vehicle for empowerment and demystification of professionalism, and by the right as an opportunity for low-cost solutions to social problems (Levick 1992). A policy driven by cost consciousness and financial pressures can apparently bring the advantages of improved life satisfaction and greater freedom (Knapp *et al.* 1992). The same mechanisms can appear to satisfy contradictory aims: 'assessment, care management and inspection are the keys to improving responses to consumer need and quality care, whilst ensuring efficient and economic use of scarce resources' (Biggs and Weinstein 1991).

This easy transition in rhetoric from cost cutting to improving quality of life is made possible partly by the chameleon-like nature of some of the core concepts underpinning the policy. Independence can be construed as better for people's self-esteem and respect; its other advantage is that people doing things for themselves costs less. Normalization requires people's integration within ordinary living networks; it is also convenient that promoting and prioritizing informal caring community networks produces less reliance on statutory services. Choice and empowerment mean people having control over their own lives; if people have the status of consumers of services, then they are responsible for the quality of those services because their demands regulate the market and they only have themselves to blame if it goes wrong. It is thus not difficult to see how community care can be constructed as both the best and the cheapest, although it is also apparent that the consensus hides deep ideological conflicts (Baldwin and Parker 1990).

Key features of the community care policy context

An analysis of the key features of the policy context follows, creating a 'community care map' to assist understanding of:

- the main policy objectives;
- the mechanisms for achieving those objectives;
- the underpinning principles.

Mixed economy of welfare

The principle of allowing market forces of supply and demand to regulate the provision of welfare services is central to community care policy. It is based on the belief that if consumers are free to choose they will use their purchasing power to regulate both price and quality in the market place by rejecting services which are not good enough or too expensive. It requires enough diversity of provision for there to be competition and choice. Increased competition between service providers should lead to improved quality and reduced cost (DoH 1990a). People who have the financial resources can purchase the care and services they require quite freely under this system. People who do not have the resources to purchase for themselves can have care and services purchased for them by the local authority, provided they have been assessed as needing it. For the local authority to undertake this role requires it to split the functions of purchase and provision of service so that, while it may purchase services from itself, it can apply the same criteria of value for money and cost-effectiveness that it would to purchase from elsewhere. Thus if better value is available elsewhere through competition in the supply side of the market, public money should, it is argued, be spent there. Guidance (DoH 1991a) defines the different roles of purchasing and providing services. Purchaser roles involve assessing the population's needs for social care, and commissioning, specifying, planning, organizing or acquiring services to meet those needs. Provider roles involve the actual delivery of services to users in line with service specifications and contracts.

In fulfilling their purchasing function local authorities must make maximum use of the independent sector (DoH 1989a). Indeed, in devolving central funding to local authorities to finance the purchase of community care services the government stipulated a key proportion to be spent in the independent sector (85 per cent in 1993–4).

The concept of a mixed economy based on supply and demand has been widely criticized. Hudson (1990) points out that the reforms are purely to one side of the equation, the supply side. In the absence of demand side reform (the government's refusal of Griffiths's proposal to subsidize individuals to make their own purchases in the market) supply side reform has had to invent concepts such as 'welfare pluralism' (extending the range and nature of suppliers) and 'internal market' (a means of engaging them in competition) to make the system work.

The application of market principles to welfare is seen as inappropriate and irrational: forces other than market forces determine demand for services (Langan 1990); services operate within a professional value system and within predetermined levels of resource, regardless of expressed consumer preference (Bamford 1990). Such a system benefits richer people and those who can articulate their demands (Baldwin and Parker 1990), who in effect will control the demand side, leaving others to go through needs assessment and rely on local authority purchase of services on their behalf. In a free market, supply will develop in response to volume of demand. In such a system it will be the needs and demands of the majority that will be met, not those of minorities whose influence in the market will be smaller (Mirza 1991). Indeed, demand will be mediated by factors additional to simple 'need': knowledge of the welfare system and of agency responsibilities, or lack of confidence in the suitability of its services, may contribute to artificially low 'demand' (Sone 1993). Additionally, there will be stigmatized groups for whom no one wants to provide, vulnerable people who cannot make demands and those who do not speak in the right way to the right people

(Victor 1991). Market forces additionally introduce economic and political uncertainty into the planning and development of services (Levick 1992) as providers concentrate on provision that is popular and profitable (Victor 1991). Such concerns contribute to suspicion of the private sector and belief in the continued role of local authorities as providers (Wistow and Hardy 1993). At most what should be envisaged is a managed market rather than a free market (Miller 1991), a vision of appropriate diversity where parties contribute to a negotiated and commonly shared plan.

Managing such a system is in itself complex, and raises a number of challenges. These have been presented (Flynn and Hurley 1993a) as purchasing dilemmas, conflicting imperatives which create a tension in the system. Purchasers, for example, require flexibility if they are to purchase services appropriate to people's individual and changing needs. Providers, however, require stability, a guaranteed demand in effect, if they are to invest in the people and structures needed to provide consistent, good quality services. What happens to innovation in service development when the guaranteed viability of tried and tested models of service is what sells well? Should purchasers control service specifications, or allow for input by providers because of their close contact with service users' changing needs? Should purchasers go to preferred regular providers, or is there room for newcomers to the market who may yet be developing the know-how to provide reliability and consistency? Should political control influence where and with whom contracts are placed? Such questions are raised but not answered by policy directives, and will take some considerable time to be addressed at a local level by the agencies concerned.

Needs-led assessment

The assessment of people's need for services is one of the local authority's key responsibilities (section 47, NHSCCA 1990) where it appears there may be a need for community care services. The local authority must then decide whether the assessed need requires the provision of community care services. Local authorities assumed these responsibilities in April 1993. It was never intended that every request for services should trigger a full assessment process. Indeed, many authorities have established a tiered eligibility structure whereby users may qualify for straightforward advice and information, standard (limited) assessment or full assessment depending on the initial level of need presented (Marchant 1993). However, when triggered, assessment should be needs-led and characterized by multidisciplinary collaboration; users and carers should be actively involved, and provided with information about available services and eligibility criteria; and assessment outcomes should inform planning about community care needs (DoH 1990a).

Needs-led assessment is one cornerstone of community care rhetoric, the basis of decisions about care (SSI 1993a). Yet 'need' in this context is construed very specifically as the requirements of individuals to enable them to achieve, maintain or restore an acceptable level of social independence or quality of life, as defined by the particular care agency or authority (DoH

1991b). While accepting that need is 'a personal concept – no two individuals will perceive or define their needs in exactly the same way' – need is expected to fall into six broad subdivisions:

- personal/social care;
- health care;
- accommodation;
- finance;
- education/employment/leisure;
- transport/access.

Definition is influenced by changes in legislation, policy and resources.

One purpose of emphasizing needs-led assessment is to move authorities away from resource-led assessment, used merely as a process for determining whether a person qualifies for an existing service (DoH 1989a). This requires a change of thinking, to frame need not in terms of residential care, day care or home help, but in terms of differing levels of assistance with personal care or daytime occupation. The objectives of intervention become the outcomes to be achieved rather than the services to be provided (Humphries 1992). The purpose is to identify the end before focusing on the means.

Accurately identifying need is thus one of the core components of assessment, but it is not the only one. What follows the definition and understanding of need is establishing eligibility for assistance and agreeing the objectives of any intervention (SSI 1993b). Inherent to assessment is the exercise of judgement about whether identified need triggers eligibility for services. It is not possible to move too far away from the influence of resource provision upon service priorities. 'Decisions on service provision will have to take account of what is available and affordable' (DoH 1989a). There is 'recognition that an assessment that demonstrates need assumes the possibility of a solution. In practice, provision may have to be resource led, and this involves setting priorities' (Centre for Policy on Ageing 1990). Thus needs-led assessment may turn out to be nothing but a disguise for resource-led assessment (Morris 1993a).

There are also fears that discrimination could arise through the local authority's power to recover some of the costs of providing services from service users themselves. Black elders, high numbers of whom are without pension eligibility and thus dependent on income support, are in a position to contribute little and thus risk being discriminated against (Jadeja and Singh 1993). This tension between the identification of need and subsequent decisions about eligibility for, and levels of, service provision led at the time of implementation to dilemmas for local authorities attempting to establish priorities which met their legal duties. Judicial review decisions, where people have challenged local authorities for not providing services they have been assessed as needing, have established that services provided under section 2 of the CSDPA 1970 could not be contingent upon finance and resource availability once an assessed need for them had been established (*R. v. Secretary of State for Education and Science, Ex parte E*, 1991; Mark Hazell, reported by Cervi and Marchant 1993). An authority without sufficient staff to perform its duties would be in breach of the Local Authority Social Services

Act 1970. The mandatory nature of this legislation regulating service provision was confirmed in 1985 (Keep 1992), while the Disabled Persons (SCR) Act 1986 established eligibility for assessment of need if requested by a disabled person or his or her carer. Section 47 of the NHSCCA 1990, in extending the local authority's duty to *assess* need far more widely, raised the expectation that large numbers of service users would be able to press for their assessed needs to be met. Guidance issued to local authorities (DoH 1992a) warns that if needs were not met legal challenges could ensue, leading to widespread speculation that local authorities would not record the outcome of assessments if they contained unmet need. Subsequent guidance (Lambert 1993) suggests that authorities could record unmet *choices* or preferences expressed by service users which fell outside the authority's eligibility criteria, and collect data on unmet *need* anonymously for service planning purposes. Legal challenges continue. The Local Commissioner for Administration (Ombudsman) ordered Tower Hamlets to compensate and reassess the needs of a service user in June 1993 after finding maladministration in failure to support him on discharge from hospital.

However, the position remains essentially unclear and subject to interpretation. For example, the Audit Commission's study of the first six months of full operation of community care in 1993 complicated the picture in commenting that counselling and advice must be offered as a service in its own right to people whose needs assessments do not lead to provision of service (Clarke 1993).

Further challenges to the concept of needs-led assessment arise from an analysis of the power balance within the assessment encounter. Despite calls for assessment to operate as a dialogue, with service users as active participants (Centre for Policy on Ageing 1990), it is, as construed in government guidance, a process led by the agency (Stevenson and Parsloe 1993). Ellis (1993) points to the implication in guidance (SSI 1991a) that, despite partnership rhetoric, the professional assessor uses a sense of superior judgement to penetrate beyond demand to actual need. While acknowledging the influence of 'differing, frequently competing perspectives on need', her study of assessment in practice leads her to conclude that the encounter is 'as much about the differential power participants have to influence the outcome'. Morris (1993a) points out that the assumption that professionals have to be in charge of the assessment process, ruling out self-assessment in case it leads to insatiable demand, is insulting and ignores evidence that service users are quite capable of rationing their use of a service if criteria are clear.

In the context of professionally led needs assessment the biases inherent in the concept of need being applied must be examined. Overtly located within an individualized dependency-led model, it is covertly influenced by white Eurocentric norms and assumptions about gendered experience. Assimilationist and culturalist policies form the basis of needs assessment in white organizations (Ahmad-Aziz *et al.* 1992), based on myths and stereotyping (Gunaratnam 1993) and leading to inappropriate services which ignore the needs of black people and their communities (NAREA undated), applying Western concepts of well-being (Mirza 1991). Unlike comparable children's legislation of the same era (CA 1989), which requires local authorities to consider a child's race, language, culture and religion, the NHS and Community Care Act 1990 is silent on these issues, making only passing comments in non-regulatory guidance (DoH 1991b) to the needs of minority ethnic groups in relation to assessment. Grimwood and Popplestone (1993) demonstrate the assumptions of a heterosexual, gender-neutral context which inform the policy context, ignoring the power dynamics within families and the pressures on women to construe their own needs as identical to those of other family members. Gender assumptions influence decisions on service delivery (Graham 1993) and result in a failure to focus services on people with the most intense needs (Bebbington and Davies 1993). Finally, concern arises about the role of established need as a passport to services. People who may *want* to enter residential care and who until 1993 had an entitlement to benefit to enable them to do so, for example, have had that right replaced by a requirement to establish *need*. The relationship between needs and rights is a complex one, and is explored further in Chapter 4.

Independence

Independence is viewed as a desirable and central goal to be attained by the provision of community care services (DoH 1989a; Centre for Policy on Ageing 1990). In this context it is construed fairly narrowly, founded on an assumption that most people want to care for themselves without assistance. The subtext of this position is that independent people have responsibility for themselves and are less likely to want to rely on state subsidized services. Any intervention by public services is aimed at supporting and facilitating individuals to feel more responsible for their own lives. Such a construction can help with what Stevenson and Parsloe (1993) see as an ideological dilemma for the government: how to establish an enterprise society which rewards individual initiative and self-advancement yet ensures adequate care for those who fail to rise to the challenge or who are its victims.

There are problems with this. The concept of independence is conflated with that of a dignified life (DoH 1990a) and presented as an uncontestable good thing, which any reasonable person would want. This in itself is an untested proposition (Goodwin 1990). Stereotyped and routinized responses can lead to inappropriate and inflexible provision, which may undermine independence as much as failing to support (Caldock 1993). People are equally institutionalized by services which restrict their community participation (Morris 1993b; Prior 1993). Indeed, Morris (1993b) proposes a much wider view that physical inability to perform daily living tasks does not inevitably create dependency, but the response of services can do so; that it is having *control* over the assistance one needs, rather than being able to manage without it, that brings independence.

Care management

Care management is defined in government guidance as 'the process of tailoring services to individual needs' (DoH, 1991b). Broad requirements specify that care management systems must:

- respond flexibly and sensitively to the needs of users and their carers;
- allow a range of options;
- intervene no more than necessary to foster independence;
- prevent deterioration;
- concentrate on those with the greatest needs.

It comprises seven core tasks:

- publishing information about the needs for which assistance is offered and the arrangements for meeting those needs;
- determining the level of assessment, matching it to the initial identified need;
- assessing need, relating needs to agency policies and priorities, and agreeing objectives for intervention;
- care planning and negotiating appropriate ways of meeting objectives;
- implementing the care plan and securing the necessary resources and services;
- monitoring, supporting and controlling the implementation of the plan;
- reviewing, reassessing need and outcomes, and revising plans where necessary.

Like many of the concepts and mechanisms in community care policy, it has acquired different meanings. As originally practised, and named 'case management', it developed as a service system response to the coordination of care (Huxley 1993), 'a way of tailoring help to meet individual need by placing responsibility for assessment and coordination with one worker or team' (Onyett 1992). Within this broad umbrella a wide variety of organizational models were identifiable, each with its own advantages and disadvantages (Renshaw 1988). Experimental schemes (Challis and Davies 1986; Davies and Challis 1986) had demonstrated the positive outcomes of needs-led case management systems on the quality, coordination and cost of services to older people. These results were highly influential on policy planning. Department of Health documents used the term 'case management', substituting 'care management' in the policy guidance (DoH 1990a) and subsequent practice guidance (DoH 1991b), along with greater emphasis on 'identifying and addressing the needs of individuals *within available resources*'. This shift in terminology facilitated the introduction of eligibility criteria to reduce spending and, like the North American term 'managed care', legitimized budget limitation in service provision (Huxley 1993). This duality of thinking is apparent in the core tasks, with the emphasis on relating need to agency policies and priorities before agreeing objectives for intervention and service plans.

Within the market economy, care management is firmly located on the purchaser side. Indeed, the clear separation of responsibility for care management from responsibility for service provision is heralded as one of the many advantages (DoH 1991b), the assumption being that care management that is divorced from provision leads to greater objectivity in decision-making and will be able to represent more effectively the interests of, and be accountable to, service users (Knapp et al. 1992). The shift of influence from those providing to those purchasing services is deliberate (DoH 1990a) and contributes to a view of care management as merely a more rational rationing system (Westland 1992).

Approaches to implementation may be categorized in a number of ways. Biggs and Weinstein (1991) identify five models:

- management models, focusing on the relationship between assessment, care planning and budget planning;
- administrative models, emphasizing budgetary planning and management;
- advocacy models, negotiating a pathway through the care system with service users;
- clinical models, involving direct therapeutic involvement with service users;
- empowerment models, focusing on community networking to change welfare systems in line with user need.

Huxley (1993) gives a more complex analysis, categorizing models by reference to their theoretical and empirical base, their primary content, their organization and their outcomes. Thus the theoretical basis can vary from an emphasis on cost-effectiveness in achieving desired welfare 'outputs' to a focus on building on strengths to achieve independence and self-determination. Primary content can be casework, assertive outreach for people refusing services, or brokerage and advocacy. Organization can follow: a clinical model, recognizing that the care manager is an important resource for the service user as a direct worker; an administrative model, which separates assessment from provision on the grounds that this promotes needs-led assessment that is less contaminated by knowledge of what is available; or a decentralized budget model, where frontline workers and managers hold the purchasing power to enable more creative local responses. Outcomes may emphasize the not necessarily compatible goals of improved service coordination, improved quality of life and improved resource distribution.

Clearly not all service users will trigger care management procedures, particularly those for whom a short-term or limited, low-cost service response is likely. Evidence exists (Challis and Davies 1993) that, from a cost-effectiveness perspective, care management should primarily be targeted on people who are otherwise likely to enter residential care, because it is more expensive than any other way of organizing service provision. Despite the government's emphasis on the split between care management and provision, evidence exists (Challis and Davies 1993) that a clinical model, in which the relationship between the care manager and the service user is an important resource, is preferable to an administrative model. This seems particularly important in the mental health field (Onyett 1992), the care manager operating less as a 'travel agent' and more as a 'travel guide'. It is here too that care management as an assertive and proactive method of involvement with 'hard to reach' service users can have positive outcomes in reduced need for inpatient care and greater user satisfaction.

Devolved budgets are seen as promoting the genuine individuation of care packages which are less constrained by existing services (Challis and Davies 1993) and as a basic prerequisite for cost consciousness because they force consideration of the relationship between needs, resources and outcomes

(Knapp *et al.* 1992), illustrating again the tension between user need and resource containment. A stringent critique of care management as envisaged in policy guidance can be made on the grounds that all its essential functions are in the hands of professionals, thus contributing to the enforced helplessness and subservience of service users (Pelikan 1991). In this analysis, care management merely reproduces the values and reality of the total institution that community care was meant to replace.

Care Programme Approach and Mental Illness Specific Grant

These are two mechanisms designed specifically to contribute towards social care provision for people with mental health problems. The Care Programme Approach is intended to ensure that systematic arrangements are made for the continuing care of people who have received psychiatric treatment. Historically, it links back to the White Paper *Better Services for the Mentally Ill* (DHSS 1975) and the circular (HC(89)5) on 'The discharge of patients from hospital' (DoH 1989b) in its emphasis on assessment, planning, coordination between services and communication with carers (Hogman 1992). It also reflects concerns about people 'falling through the net' (Schneider 1993), the drift of people with mental health problems into homelessness or the criminal justice system, and high rates of readmission in psychiatric hospital linked to poor community provision. Outlined in circulars (HC(90)23, LAC(90)11; DoH 1990b), the approach requires collaboration between health and local authorities to plan and provide for the social care needs of people referred to specialist psychiatric services, as either outpatients or inpatients, and empowers local authorities to continue to expand social care services to people being treated in the community 'as resources allow'. A key feature is intended to be the involvement of users and carers in the planning of care programmes.

The Mental Illness Specific Grant (HC(90)24, LAC(90)10; DoH 1990c) is intended to encourage local authorities to expand their social care provision in this field. It is a ring-fenced amount within community care funding (section 50, NHSCCA 1990), financing up to 70 per cent of the cost of additional services, the local authority itself contributing 30 per cent. Schemes so funded can be for social care of any kind agreed between the health and local authorities, to contribute towards the needs of people whose mental ill-health is so severe that they have been accepted for treatment by psychiatric services, or would benefit from such services.

There have been major delays in the implementation of the Care Programme Approach, variously attributed (Hogman 1992; Schneider 1993) to the lack of any detailed guidance, an absence of new resources and confusion about its relationship both with after-care (section 117, MHA 1983) and with care management. It has become increasingly clear that its application to all service users is resisted by professionals and some users, and that there are considerable barriers to planning in partnership with users and carers without major review of existing decision-making structures and mechanisms (North *et al.* 1993). Additionally, the government's review of mental health legislation, conducted during 1993, recommended a 'supervised discharge' power under which former patients may be subject to a treatment plan, involving the appointment of a key worker, a requirement to live at a specified place and attend for medical treatment, training or occupation, and grant access to professional staff. This approach contains elements of both the Care Programme Approach and Guardianship (section 7, MHA 1983), and could replace both in respect of some mental health service users.

Greater haste has been apparent in local authorities' use of the Mental Illness Specific Grant, with evidence of rapid and innovative development, particularly in day care (DoH 1993a). Concerns have been expressed about the quality of services funded in this way and a lack of systematic consultation with users, carers and potential providers, particularly from black communities and organizations (Hogman 1992). Expenditure by local authorities on mental health services is highly variable, and monitoring (Stone 1992) demonstrates a reduction of overall resourcing levels because of cuts in local authorities' base budgets. Considerable concern remains about levels of investment in after-care facilities (DoH 1994).

Contracts

The purchaser–provider split has generated a number of mechanisms for regulating the transactions which lead to service provision. A *service specification* bridges assessment of need, whether for individuals or groups, and the purchase of service. It is a statement about how a social services department requires a particular service to be delivered (Whitfield and Stewart 1991) and will focus on the objectives and outcomes alongside the practicalities of inputs, processes and outputs. The specification forms the basis either for the local authority's own services provided in-house, or for negotiating a contract to purchase services from an external provider. *Contracts* confirm an agreement by a purchaser to trade and commission services from a provider (Whitfield and Stewart 1991). A process of negotiation will determine the contribution to be made by the provider in relation to the service specification, and will result in the contract specification and contract conditions which spell out the mutual responsibilities of the respective parties. Various terminologies reflect the differing relationships between the parties: service contract, service agreement, partnership agreement and grant arrangements all denote contracts, but reflect varying degrees of trust and flexibility. Government guidance (DoH 1991d) recommends different types of contracts for differing situations, with variations in the degree of flexibility in the arrangements specified.

Contracts can be used in a variety of purchasing arrangements (Whitfield and Stewart 1993): *block contracts*, which purchase access to facilities rather than services for a specific number, and have the advantage of economies of scale but restrict flexibility and competition; *price-by-case contracts*, which specify a cost of each individual use of the service, allowing greater flexibility and choice, but at a higher cost because of the risk of low volume; and *cost and volume contracts*, which allow for a specified volume of service at a specified total cost, and thus offer some security on volume while preserving the possibility of choice.

One of the key requirements of contracting for community care is cost-effectiveness (DoH 1989a). Value for money is an associated and often quoted term. Both imply a preoccupation with limiting financial expenditure by attempting to place a value on factors, such as quality of life, which are both intangible and subject to highly subjective interpretation. An additional factor in this equation is the element of choice for service users, intended to be exercised after assessment in relation to the means chosen for meeting the needs prioritized. The form of contracting arrangements favoured by the local authority could severely limit that choice if only a 'fixed menu' can be offered, because resources are tied up in contracts for a single type of provision, or from one provider. Flynn and Hurley (1993b) advocate a range of more flexible conditions within contracts, such as specifying outcome rather than the method by which it is to be achieved, leaving the service user free to negotiate this with the provider.

Research results have prompted concerns that contracts limit innovation, increase bureaucracy and fail to increase user choice and involvement. The professionals assessing need and allocating resources still retain control over choices (Common and Flynn 1992). Voluntary organizations are concerned that they will lose their independent advocacy role by being 'owned' under local authority contracts rather than the independent recipient of grants (Langan 1990) and that their developmental role will suffer by having to concentrate on what is established and therefore marketable (Lewis 1993). This problem is particularly acute for black voluntary groups, for whom being asked to act as 'agents' under contract to the local authority's white power compromises the very qualities that make them acceptable and attractive to the users of their services (Dourado 1991).

Carers

Reliance on informal care networks is an integral part of community care policy, accompanied by an assumption that this is acceptable (Baldwin and Parker 1990) and indeed desirable. Support for carers is a high priority, reflecting growing evidence about the consequences of a caring role. Carers are to be involved as full partners in the assessment and care management process, and have the right to ask for their own separate assessment if the care plan does not adequately address their own needs (DoH 1990a).

The General Household Survey (1985) identified 6 million people involved in caring tasks. Further secondary analysis gave a fuller picture, finding approximately 1.8 million people undertaking substantial amounts of care, the rest offering 'help' of varying degrees (Lawton and Parker 1993). Trends in the experience of people substantially involved in caring include:

- a loss of income and restricted employment opportunities;
- impact on physical health;
- a lack of privacy, loss of freedom and role conflict, particularly for women;
- an uneasy relationship with agencies, who see carers both as resources to be maximized and as people in need of supported well-being;

- a low likelihood of receiving services in their own right;
- their 'cared for' person being less likely to receive services if the carer lives in the same household;
- gender differences in the response of agencies, with domiciliary support being more likely to be given where men are the main users.

These impacts may well be experienced differentially. Black carers have, for instance, experienced neglect from statutory agencies, or inappropriate and restricted services with little attention to the structural disadvantage and racism compounding their task (McCalman 1990; Gunaratnam 1993). The increasing reliance on informal networks intensifies inequalities experienced by women and the exploitation of their labour (Baldwin and Twigg 1991), in terms both of gender roles amounting to 'compulsory altruism' (Land 1991) within family networks and of women's involvement in the proliferation of 'paid volunteer' schemes (Baldock and Ungerson 1991). In this analysis the reliance for effective community care on what is seen as a profoundly sexist institution, the family, had led to calls for expansion rather than retraction of institutional care or the development of other forms of collective care (Finch 1984; Dalley 1988). A counter view (Morris 1991/2) explores how such conclusions can be profoundly disablist in assuming that to avoid the oppression of one group of people, non-disabled women, it is legitimate to oppress disabled women and men by advocating their confinement in institutional care.

In a further contribution to the debate about gender issues in community care provision, Baldwin and Twigg (1991) examine the evidence for gender divisions in caring. Men are more commonly involved in caring than is often supposed, particularly where they are acting as the main carer to a spouse, but the care of non-spousal dependents falls predominantly to women. Women are more likely to be undertaking intimate and time-consuming caring tasks for which support is not often forthcoming from relatives, friends and neighbours. Arber and Gilbert (1993) similarly note wide diversity within caring situations, proposing that men are more likely to 'drift' into caring through the existence of a prior relationship with either a spouse or a parent in whose house they still live; women are more likely to become involved in an elective caring situation, such as when a vulnerable parent moves in.

Such varied experiences, and the 'mixture of love, a sense of duty and lack of choice' which brings many carers to caring (Keith 1990), have produced sustained pressure for recognition of carers' contributions, the creation of flexible and responsive services, with opportunities for respite, practical help and attention to emotional needs. Consultation and information about services are also seen as key factors, together with better attention to the needs of black carers and access to income and employment opportunities. The prioritization of practical support for carers as one of the key community care objectives (DoH 1989a), together with provision in subsequent guidance for consultation and for carers' needs and choices to be taken into account, provides a framework which at least legitimates carers' interests, if at the cost of consolidating their involvement in community care.

Planning

Local authorities are responsible for publishing a plan for the provision of community care services in their area (section 46, NHSCCA 1990), in consultation with health authorities, family health services authorities, local housing authorities, voluntary agencies representing users and carers, and voluntary resource providers. The purposes of this requirement are to encourage local authorities to plan strategically for their new responsibilities, to ensure that planning is undertaken in collaboration with other agencies and to communicate proactively and clearly with the local population (DoH 1989a). Plans should cover a three-year period, but be reviewed and updated annually. The content of the plan must include:

• assessment of the needs of the local population;
• strategic objectives for community care implementation;
• intentions for gathering information required for planning purposes;
• assessment and care management arrangements for individuals;
• organization and management of purchasing role;
• improvements to domiciliary and carers' services;
• coordination with health authorities and other agencies;
• information available to users and carers about services;
• staff training;
• how the independent sector contribution is to be stimulated;
• quality assurance and service standards systems, including complaints procedures.

Local authorities were required to publish their first plans by April 1992. Wistow *et al.* (1993) found considerable variation in the amount of consultation undertaken with various stakeholders. Voluntary agencies, the independent residential sector and carers' groups have all complained of less consultation than they would have wished (Clode 1992a). Plans were, where possible, to be jointly produced with health authorities, or, at least, to complement those of health authorities. Although many were jointly issued, there was little evidence of detailed negotiation and decision-making on roles and relationships between agencies. The requirement that plans be presented in a form accessible to the local population produced variable results. Wistow *et al.* conclude that the early plans were more focused on aims and objectives than on resources for achieving them or mechanisms for performance evaluation and review. Questions remain over the wide and varied functions served by the publication of plans. More effective consultation mechanisms at local levels, both with service users and between agencies, must be evolved.

Seamless service

Community care policy (DoH 1989a) is founded on the premise that a person's health care needs, which should be provided for by the health authority, can be distinguished from his or her social care needs, which are the responsibility of the local authority. This distinction governs the funding arrangements of the respective agencies and necessitates the emphasis upon joint working to provide a 'seamless service'. Health authorities must liaise with social services departments to arrange social care provision for patients and social services must ensure that primary and community health provision is included in care packages (DoH 1989a). The objective is service provision in which the boundaries between primary health care, secondary health care and social care do not form barriers seen from the perspective of the service user (DoH 1990a). Poor coordination between agencies was one of the main concerns of the Audit Commission's original report (1986), with subsequent calls for clearer definitions of the distinctions between the services (Audit Commission 1992). Subsequent evidence fails to demonstrate real improvement (Bebbington and Charnley 1990; SSI 1992a). The complex reasons for poor collaboration are explored in more detail in Chapter 8. There are, however, some influential policy level factors.

First, the distinction between health care and social care is arguably a false one, the boundaries being difficult to draw (Centre for Policy on Ageing 1990). People's needs do not always fall into neat administrative divisions. For instance, social factors contribute to the development of mental health problems, and people with mental ill-health have a range of social care needs that are bound up with their health status (Huxley 1990), such that for maximum effectiveness health and social care services should be accessed singly and delivered together (Goldberg and Huxley 1992). Research into community care implementation has demonstrated that 'the idea that people can be neatly divided into those who have clinical problems and present those to health services, and those who have social problems, and present them to social services, is clearly untenable' (Huxley *et al.* 1993). Indeed, the split may have more to do with the organization and grouping of professional skills and thinking than with user need, a by-product of professional power (Wilding 1982).

Second, there is speculation that the blurred distinction between health and social care is an important contributory factor in a gradual if undeclared shift from health services which are free at the point of delivery to social care services which are means tested, with access regulated by strict need assessment. This problem is particularly apparent in community care for frail older people (Rickford 1993), where financial responsibility can be shunted between agencies by a paper exercise of redefining people's needs as being for social rather than health care. The reverse scenario is also possible, with care managers juggling budgets tempted to steer people towards health care provision.

Third, the picture is made infinitely more complex by the developing internal market in the health service. Clode (1992b) considers the impact of the creation of hospital trusts (providers), identifying dangers that inpatient services could be inappropriately prioritized in order to preserve income, or that any community services developed could be inappropriately dominated by medical model thinking. Long-stay hospitals' status as opt-out trusts could cut across both the hospital closure programme and the policy of local authorities having a lead role in community care services (Values into Action 1992). Indeed, there is evidence that such hospitals are contracting directly with health authorities to continue providing services of a social care nature (Values into Action 1993a).

Organizational structures and responsibilities are still developing. Joint purchasing by social services departments and health authorities can create consortia big enough to put pressure on providers to conform to agreed service patterns. The role of general practitioners as purchasers of care is still evolving, both in terms of the purchasing power of FHSAs jointly with DHAs and in terms of their power to purchase social care through their own fundholding practices. Conversely, there are suggestions (Wistow 1993) that local authorities could develop a role as purchasers of health care.

Achieving a seamless service between health care and social care provision clearly requires more than government exhortation to work in partnership. Until organizational and structural clarity is achieved, service users presenting multiple needs may well continue to experience poorly coordinated services.

Consumerism

The rhetoric of community care policy presents people who need social care services as 'consumers', able to choose freely in the market place and thus determine both their own use of services and, through the forces of supply and demand, the development of 'quality products'. 'The rationale for this reorganisation is the empowerment of users and carers . . . this redressing of the balance of power is the best guarantee of a continuing improvement in the quality of services' (DoH 1991e).

The principles of consumerism underpin many of the key mechanisms within community care provision. Services are meant to be *accessible*, in terms of both geographical proximity and user friendliness. People should have *information* about what is on offer and the mechanisms devised to determine eligibility. They may use this information to exercise *choice*, which underlies all the government's proposals (DoH 1989a), and a right to *redress*, for example through complaints procedures. There must be mechanisms for *representation* and consultation, to enable views to be expressed and exert an influence on the processes of planning (DoH 1991f).

Fundamental to this construction is the emphasis on user involvement and participation in all the processes of assessment and decision-making. The notion of participation develops into that of a partnership between professionals and service users (DoH 1991b) and between the various agencies involved (DoH 1990a). Professionals must thus change from being expert definers of need and rationers of services, to being resources which service users can negotiate to use as required (SSI 1993b) and to working with users of services and their relatives in ways which ensure that information is properly shared, options are considered and, whenever possible, users are closely involved in the decisions which affect their lives (SSI 1993a).

There are, however, problems with the attempt to build welfare policy on the notion of consumerism. First, there are fundamental differences between the endeavours of commercial enterprise and public welfare (Pfeffer and Coote 1991). Public welfare deals in need, not want. A necessary consequence of its primary purpose of reducing disadvantage is that all who have needs should receive, regardless of their purchasing power in the market. Consumerism and customer care ideologies in welfare do little to promote rights of citizenship or to respond to collective need (Hambleton and Hoggett 1990). The key principles all have dubious application in the field of public welfare.

Accessibility is compromised by eligibility criteria and thresholds of need that must be established before even assessment is available. *Information* as a means of empowering people to choose is highly dependent upon what information is given and how (Coote 1992) and can be restricted by professionals as a means of controlling demand (Lewis 1991). Service users do not consider the information they receive about provision to be adequate (SSI 1992a). Some groups of users have more difficulty than others in accessing the information they need (Allen *et al.* 1993).

Choice is constrained by several factors, especially the limited availability of resources. The notion that the supply of services will increase in response to demand is patently flawed in a cash-limited service (Williamson 1993). Even where budgets are devolved to care managers there are strict resource limits to be worked to. The standard service range of domiciliary services inadequately meets the needs of people who might choose to use more intensive and extensive services were they available (Challis *et al.* 1988). What is available has often been determined by top-down preconceived ideas of what is suitable and appropriate (Humphries 1992). Thus service users find that there is duplication – services that are easily available from both the local authority and informal community support networks – and gaps that no one wants to fill (Morris 1993b). A further constraint on choice is how the local authority operates its purchase of service arrangements: both block contracts and cost and volume contracts contribute towards a fixed menu provision rather than freedom of choice for service users. The concept of needs assessment inevitably limits choice: residential care for those not assessed as needing it is only a choice for those who have the personal means to pay (Biggs 1990). This situation derives from the original impetus of the Audit Commission (1985) in recommending that expensive residential care should be restricted to those who most need it, rather than 'optional' users.

Representation is similarly limited as a mechanism for consumer power in public welfare. There is an inevitable mismatch between the image of a consumer with money to spend and the reality of disempowered and discriminated-against groups (Cornwell 1992/3). The attempt to reconstruct the previously disempowered and institutionalized patient as an independent consumer in a free market society is flawed (Prior 1993) because the rhetoric of consumerism does not transform the power relationships between professionals and service users. Assessment, despite users' representation, remains firmly within the professional domain, to the extent that some users and carers remain unaware that it has taken place (SSI 1993c). Even service users' choices are subject to professional vetting: options should be fully discussed with users and carers and where possible genuine choice should be offered, but practitioners must satisfy themselves that the option selected is that most suited to the identified need (DoH 1991b). Moreover, representation in a free market favours the advocacy of more powerful people over the voices of others whose needs may be as great but whose demands are less vociferously made.

Redress in this system is limited. A true consumer, if dissatisfied, is free not to purchase or to go elsewhere. Professional power in the context of needs assessment makes these unlikely choices for service users who could be subject to compulsion if their 'choices' place them at risk, or where alternatives quite simply do not exist. There is little attention in government guidance to situations where people refuse desperately needed services because they feel they cannot afford to pay the assessed charge (Stevenson and Parsloe 1993) or to the implications of care management for 'involuntary' users of services (Fisher 1990a). For many, redress for inadequacy in provision will come too late, the consequences having already been suffered in sometimes life-threatening ways (Pfeffer and Coote 1991). For others there can be no redress for the treatment received in the context of statutory provision. 'To me, the administration of a large dose of major tranquilliser, and the physical manhandling [*sic*] that accompanied it, remains a sharp reminder that I have neither the respect, power, nor legal protection of any consumer' (Plumb 1987).

Such experiences contribute to the conclusion that, like many users of community care, 'survivors of the mental health system are no more consumers of mental health services than cockroaches are consumers of Rentokil' (Barker and Peck 1987). Thus, consumerism applied to welfare sits in an uneasy relationship with factors which constrain and limit its relevance. In the absence of radical reform to give service users true purchasing power, it is the local authority as purchaser which retains the power to influence the market (Victor 1991).

There is in effect a fundamental confusion of two separate agendas: one derived from a merger of commercial and consumerist interests in which agencies seek to involve service users in a dialogue which will produce desirable and profitable services; the other derived from the self-advocacy movement's agenda of empowerment in the sense of people achieving a greater degree of control over their lives. The politics of liberation sit uncomfortably with those of the market place (Croft and Beresford 1990). The confusion of buying power with empowerment (Ramon 1991b) masks the sleight of hand by which service users remain essentially at the mercy of both professional discretion and profit motives in the market.

Quality

Quality has become a much used term in welfare provision. The policy of community care is meant to improve the quality of care available to service users. The local authority is central in determining and monitoring the quality of what is provided (DoH 1989a). Yet multiple pressures on social services departments make the questions 'what is quality?' and 'what are the most appropriate arrangements for its delivery?' challenging ones (DoH 1992b). Pfeffer and Coote (1991) identify various ways in which the term quality is used. Quality has traditionally implied a superior, and probably expensive, product, ownership of which conveys prestige and status. A scientific approach to quality measures conformity to standards of acceptability as defined by 'experts': how fit for its purpose a product is. A managerial approach has a 'mission' of being the best at satisfying customers' requirements in order to pursue and maintain a market advantage. A consumerist approach sees quality as achieved by empowering customers to exert an influence on providers, through acting together to lobby for change, or through individually seeking representation and redress. These models give rise to mechanisms for pursuing quality, from setting performance indicators and service standards characteristic of the scientific approach, through the total quality management rhetoric of the managerial approach, which aims for commitment to quality to be embedded in all levels of the organization, to the provisions for complaints, redress and representation characteristic of consumerist approaches.

Mechanisms for ensuring quality in community care services reflect a mixture of most of these approaches. The consumerist interest is strongly represented by the requirement that local authorities establish procedures for hearing representations, including complaints, from service users (section 50, NHSCCA 1990).

Complaints procedures should (DoH 1990a):

- provide an effective means of allowing service users or their representatives to complain about the quality or nature of social services;
- ensure that complaints are acted on;
- aim to resolve complaints quickly and as close to the point of service delivery as is acceptable and appropriate;
- give those denied a service an accepted means of challenging the decision made;
- provide in defined circumstances for the independent review of a complaint;
- give managers and councillors an additional means of monitoring performance and the extent to which service objectives are being achieved.

Accessibility of the procedures to users and carers is prioritized, together with the need for all departmental staff to develop an awareness and understanding of what is required by them (DoH 1991g). Incorporating and prioritizing service user definitions of quality and satisfaction is strongly emphasized (DoH 1992b). Requirements for representation from and involvement of user groups in the planning processes also reflect the consumerist approach.

Other mechanisms derive more directly from the managerial approach, with an emphasis on quality assurance which encompasses organizational procedures that aim to ensure that concern for quality is designed and built in to services, demonstrated by an explicit statement of policy setting out agency expectations and standards and systematic and comprehensive arrangements to ensure the required standards are achieved (DoH 1991d). The requirement for community care plans to be published and the power of the Secretary of State to issue directions and guidance over the full range of personal social services activities by local authorities (DoH 1989a) are part of the quality assurance endeavour. The setting of standards in itself reflects the scientific approach, and leads into quality control mechanisms, the 'processes of verification [which] will include systematic monitoring, recurring and one-off audit activity designed to establish whether standards are being achieved' (DoH 1991d).

The concept of setting standards, which meet the requirements of the purchaser and service user and to which the provider is committed, is central to the government's view of quality in community care (DoH 1990a). Pfeffer and Coote (1991) point out that the Social Services Inspectorate has increasingly moved to evaluating local authority services against standard measures. A related development has been the introduction into service provision agencies of an adapted version of the British Standards Institute measure BS5750, derived from manufacturing, which measures the quality of an organization by reference to whether the services (products) it provides are fit for their purpose and poses the question of whether the service is designed and delivered in such a way as to satisfy customer need (DoH 1992b).

One important quality control mechanism in community care is the arm's-length inspection unit which local authorities are required to set up (section 48, NHSCCA 1990) to inspect both public and private residential care against common standards, and to regulate standards in other services such as domiciliary provision. Inspection units, from April 1991, have been required (DoH 1990a) to:

- evaluate the quality of care provided and the quality of life experienced in private and voluntary residential care homes and in local authority establishments similarly providing board and personal care;
- ensure that a consistent approach is taken to inspection of public, private and voluntary provision;
- respond to the demands and opportunities for quality control created by the growth in contracted-out service provision;
- undertake their duties even-handedly, efficiently and cost-effectively.

There are, however, some problems associated with the approach to quality envisaged by community care policies. First, while government guidance envisages that measures such as inspection are consistent with a quality assurance approach (DoH 1991h), the two do not always sit easily together. Inspection is often experienced negatively both by those carrying it out and by those being inspected (Raynes 1993). This is partly attributable to the differing expectations staff may have of this activity. The SSI (1993a) maintains the importance of balancing regulation and freedom to provide innovative and responsive services, a tension which has resulted in wide inconsistencies in how inspection units are carrying out their work (Witton 1992). There are certainly risks in locating an authority's prime quality assurance role solely in inspection: risks that the role conflict is irreconcilable, that development work is resisted because it is associated with inspection, and that quality assurance becomes an isolated rather than an integrated function (DoH 1992b). Even as a quality control mechanism, inspection has its pitfalls. Its coverage of community care services, for example, is partial. There is no duty to register and inspect private domiciliary service agencies, despite the intensive and intimate levels of care they may be providing. This gap and the government's resistance to legislation have led to the development of voluntary accreditation schemes which will at least guarantee minimum standards. There are additional problems associated with inspecting services which offer intangible quality benefits, such as 'independence' or 'dignity'. Gibbs and Sinclair (1992) found little agreement between inspectors of older people's residential homes on their overall judgement of a home, or indeed on the basic values to be applied and the indicators for them. Even where indicators can be agreed, the danger exists that they encourage the measurement and evaluation of activity rather than outcome (Onyett 1992) and result in a checklist or tick-box mentality in which it cannot be guaranteed that the parts add up to the desired whole.

A second problem relates to the assumption that it is the responsibility of the purchaser of services to define and specify quality in contracts and that the provider's role is to conform to what is specified under the purchasing agreement. This may be feasible for tangible elements of the service, but pays little attention to the notion of adding value through the quality of relationship between the provider and service user. It also limits users' input to whatever they have been able successfully to negotiate at the assessment stage, rather than making their perspective integral to the whole process of assessing quality. Such an assumption also begs the question of who is responsible when a service, seen from the perspective of the service user, is of poor quality. It will be tempting for purchasers to assume that providers have somehow failed their side of the contract, whereas the problem might equally be with the assessment, the care planning, service specification or contracting processes.

A third problem derives from a confusion of terms and concepts between quality in service provision and quality of life. Quality in community care rhetoric is overtly used to describe both 'a commitment to highest standards of service provision and services [that are] underpinned by a commitment to quality of life' (SSI 1992a). To some extent this assumes that 'the community' is somehow intrinsically therapeutic and that integration with it would occur spontaneously if services were located outside segregated institutions (Ramon 1991a). The evidence does not always support this. While community-based placements have been established which offer much richer social and material environments than the hospitals they replace (Mansell and Beasley 1993), it is also the case that some people end up living in circumstances that are just as institutional as those of the hospital environment (Prior 1993). People may be *in* the community but are not *of* the community. For quality of service provision to be directly related to quality of life requires a greater emphasis upon the self-definition and self-advocacy of service users as contributors towards defining the requirements that will ensure that one leads to the other. Pfeffer and Coote (1991) propose a different conceptual frame for quality in public service provision, a 'democratic approach' which borrows from other approaches the concepts of fitness for purpose, responsiveness and consumer empowerment, but locates them within a primary goal of equality. Strategies for ensuring quality within this model will include a focus on open information and decision-making systems, the identification of rights and effective channels for public participation, as well as systematic auditing using specifications negotiated with the public, and methods of review which take account of users' needs and experiences.

Such an approach is endorsed by development work that has been undertaken to identify effective quality assurance mechanisms in local authorities, in which responsiveness to service user views and a focus on the point of interaction with service users are two key characteristics of a robust quality assurance system (DoH 1992b). The emphasis in such an approach to quality will move away from standard 'scientific' measures towards varied definitions which can reflect the diversity of communities, not only who use services but who might use services, so that the accessibility, appropriateness, adequacy and accountability of services are no longer defined by reference to a white dominant majority (Mirza 1991). The focus of a quality of life dimension in quality assurance is much wider than merely upon services provided. It amounts to a new 'quality paradigm' which engages with the wider environments that shape people's experience and uses qualitative, value-led, user-based measures to judge whether policies for quality assurance are having the desired impact on people's lives (Hudson 1991).

Conclusion

From this analysis of the objectives, mechanisms and underpinning principles of community care policy two broad themes emerge which contain unresolved tensions. These tensions, however, are not merely differences of opinion over fine detail; they are conflicting views of the world informed by political ideology and core human values, and as such unlikely to be easily resolved. Their relevance here is that their existence at a policy and conceptual level is manifested at an individual and practice level in daily challenges, both of understanding and of action.

The first centres on debates about the state's role in relation to the personal welfare of its citizens. The transition to the policy of community care in many ways represents a transition from welfare state to state welfare, a shift of perspective from universal state paternalism emphasizing care and protection to selective residual provision for those unable to survive through individualistic self-provision. Carried with this transition is reinforcement of the concept of need as a passport to state involvement, and a side-stepping of the issue of rights to services. Rights, where they are implied by the rhetoric of choice, are those of consumers, rather than those of citizenship. The needs/rights debate, and the influence of resources upon what emerges in legislation and policy, are discussed in Chapter 4.

The second underlying theme contains debates about the primary purpose of community care, reflecting different beliefs about whether need arises from individual pathology or from social conditions. The cosy image of vulnerable individuals having their needs assessed and met by care packages of appropriate and accessible services implies that social care's primary purpose is to help people compensate for and adjust to, rather than change, their experience of society. Images of disability with which legislation is imbued (Braye and Preston-Shoot 1992a), for example, reflect the stereotyped and patronizing views of vulnerability and dependency. These are being challenged by a self-advocacy movement, demonstrating the greater disabling effects that derive from social and structural factors in society than from impairment. Yet the community care blueprint ignores, or assumes as favourable, the wider environmental context of service users' experience (Wilson 1992). Integration within a community is often more influenced by the availability of housing, education and employment, yet community care service agencies have little influence here (Knapp 1993). Community care may change the *location* of the service, but does little to redefine the assumptions on which the service is based, models of care that emphasize individual pathology merely being translated from one setting to another. Thus, for example, discharge from psychiatric hospital does not mean freedom from psychiatric control (Bean and Mounser 1993). This theme will be explored further in the context of power and empowerment in Chapter 5.

Why has community care had the apparent support it has enjoyed, if it is concealing such a deep division of ideology and belief? One explanation is that the concept is sufficiently wide to be able to accommodate the different meanings and significance bestowed upon it. The term can be as appealing to those advocating ordinary, non-institutional living as to those concerned with cost containment. Service user empowerment is attractive both to those who believe consumer power to be the key to quality in the mixed market and to those who want, or support others in having, greater autonomy and control over their lives. Thus consensus can successfully mask conflict, and prevent the debates from taking place.

Exercise 1.1.   Think about the agency for which you work, or one of which you have had some experience. How does it fit within the structure of community care? What is its place in the mixed market? What is your role within that?

Exercise 1.2.   Who are the people who use the services of the agency you have in mind? How does the agency communicate with those people? How easy do those people find it to have their views heard by the agency?

Exercise 1.3.   How would you define quality within the function of the agency you have in mind? How do you think other people would define it – users, staff, managers? How would you know, if you were trying to evaluate the agency's functioning, that it had achieved quality? What would you see, hear, think, feel?

2 Values in

social care

The analysis in Chapter 1 of the policy foundations for social care illustrated that the legislative framework is highly influential on the social care task. Law and policy are, however, only one part of the story. They reflect political intentions which are derived from a set of beliefs about 'the right way' to provide for people's needs. These beliefs in turn express principles that are collectively 'valued' and embedded within society's structure and functioning. Additionally, individuals hold their own personal value systems, which will define and influence how they think and act. This will contribute to how they interpret the legal and policy mandate for their professional tasks.

Values are influential at every level. Collectively they give form and meaning to a culture, serving to differentiate it from another (Harris 1991). Individually they are the grounds, explicit or implicit, on which people make decisions (Fairbairn and Fairbairn 1987). In the professional arena they govern what practitioners think they *ought* to do, as opposed to what they want to or can do, and they give rise to standards and obligations (CCETSW 1976).

Timms (1983) gives a wide definition of values as 'any kind of belief and obligation, anything preferred for any reason or for no apparent reason, any objective in the short or the long run, any ideal or rule'. He stresses the importance of distinguishing between *economic value* and *values*, and differentiates between quantitative value (what something is worth), attributive value (value ascribed to something) and underlying value (belief which causes us to value some things above others). In the professional arena values become translated into ethical imperatives and are thus concerned with professional *conscience*, that which *should* be done from a moral perspective, following convictions as to what is right. The concept of values in social care thus represents a complex amalgamation of professional ethics, political beliefs and personal morality (Shardlow 1989).

Why are values important in social care? There is increasing consensus that focusing on the knowledge and skills that workers bring to the task gives only a partial picture, since personal and professional values filter what is seen and the sense made of it, and shape purposes, beliefs and action. There is no such thing as value-free work, only workers who have not stopped to think what their values are (Mullender and Ward 1991). Even the sources of knowledge upon which social care practice is based are socially constructed, determined by societal values (Williams 1993). In terms of individual decision-making, knowledge alone does not identify what workers *should* do when faced with choices between alternative courses of action (Horne 1987). Decisions in such dilemmas are inevitably value-led. In this context values are a safeguard: where professionals hold powers on behalf of society there should be a set of principles which govern how that power is exercised, and guidance on how to act in complex, often conflictual situations (Shardlow 1989). In short, values are important because they are located at every strategic point in the exercise of professional responsibility, from how workers construe its meaning through to the techniques they use (Timms 1983).

If values are so fundamental, they must be articulated and debated in the same way that the legislative framework has been. Their impact must be acknowledged and questioned. There are dangers in assuming a common-sense consensus about what is valued (Biehal and Sainsbury 1991) or in placing too much trust in professional objectivity. Practitioners can 'harbour the mistaken belief they are being professional and objective, when in reality they are making assessments and decisions based on their cultural values' (Harris 1991). Even where there is a bottom line assumption about acceptable and unacceptable, on which the state's power to intervene is based, it is essential to analyse assumptions and be aware of profound social and personal subjectivity involved in the assessment of other people's lives (Stevenson 1989). Ramon (1991b) identifies the potential danger of not opening up a values discourse: the more taken for granted a value is, the more powerful it becomes in terms of its hold over people's views and actions because it is less open for consideration. Value talk can thus become disguised as factual discourse, and used to justify action when it should only inform (Cheetham 1989). Clearly articulated values and principles can make positive contributions to social care practice, helping to reduce ambiguity and clarify priorities (Knapp *et al.* 1992) for policy-makers, managers and practitioners alike.

What values are important in social care? Two broad categories may be identified, each with its own distinct and at times mutually exclusive characteristics. On the one hand are values located in a long tradition of social care. These urge practitioners to 'treat people better' in the context of allotted roles and place in the social structure. On the other hand are values calling for radical change to, and renegotiation of, existing roles and social structures, to create a fairer society. Thus the traditional agenda is to bring about the adjustment of service users to existing conditions in society, a focus on 'personal' problems. The radical agenda emphasizes the structural context in which problems are produced and reproduced (Rojek *et al.* 1988). Within these broad categories, particularly the former, several variations and

Table 2.1   Values in social care

Traditional	Radical
Respect for persons	Citizenship
Paternalism and protection	Participation
Normalization and social role valorization	Community presence
Equality of opportunity	Equality
Anti-discriminatory practice	Anti-oppressive practice
Partnership	Empowerment, user control

subtleties can be identified. These will be explored as distinct themes (see Table 2.1).

Traditional values

Respect for persons

'Implicit in the practice of social care in residential, day, community or domiciliary settings is the recognition of the dignity and value of every human being' (Social Care Association 1988). People who use social care services are to be valued for their unique individuality, and respected in their exercise of autonomy. Consensus is assumed about individual moral rights, expressed as broad concepts such as 'achieving personal potential' and 'being true to one's own beliefs' (Centre for Policy on Ageing 1984). Practitioners are urged to respect users' privacy, to observe confidentiality, to value people's individual capabilities and to promote choice and independence as routes to personal fulfilment.

These concepts, linked together in a values package comprising the core components of privacy, dignity, independence, choice, rights and fulfilment, have been promoted widely in official guidance on the essential foundations of good quality care (DoH 1989c), standards against which it will be judged (DoH 1990d) and aids to decision-making in dilemmas about risk and protection (SSI 1993d). Professional literature exploring the tasks of both purchasers and providers of social care is peppered with references to respect for persons, privacy, dignity and individualization as determinants of practice (see, for example, Rogers 1990; Orme and Glastonbury 1993), and emphasizes the uniqueness of the individual (Kitwood and Bredin 1992).

This value system draws on a tradition of prioritizing the quality of relationship between 'helper' and 'helped', which, though deriving from social casework, has generalized to the interactive processes of social care. Key work here was that of Biestek (1957), who saw the relationship as 'the soul of social casework . . . through it flow the mobilisation of the capacities of the individual and the mobilisation of community resources'. Biestek constructed a set of principles to be observed in helping: individualization, acceptance, non-judgementalism, self-determination and confidentiality. He saw these as prerequisites for a process of change and development in the user, a view based on the assumption that contact with the helping agency stems from personal deficit, which can be remedied. What he describes essentially as *processes* have, however, become reified into *values* to be observed by practitioners. Developed by others (for example, Hollis 1970), they have had considerable impact on professional practice and now appear, sometimes under different terminology but essentially the same, in government guidance and contemporary literature.

The value base emphasizing respect for persons has not survived without criticism. First, the terminology used to describe such values as self-determination, dignity and choice is very broad and non-specific (Timms 1989), occasioning a wide range of meaning and interpretation, with little agreement as to what they mean as guidelines for practice (Horne 1987). Second, the usefulness of such concepts, not just as moral statements but also as operational principles, is difficult to sustain in everyday practice, which is influenced by competing imperatives such as resource constraint (Sainsbury 1989), and where agency authority functions and statutory requirements limit the extent to which consistency with broad principles can be maintained (Horne 1987). Third, their status is unclear. Is 'acceptance' an attitude, a technique or an outcome? Is 'self-determination' an end or a means to an end? Is 'respect for persons' a behaviour, principle or aim (Timms 1983)? Such ambiguity contributes to the difficulty of making a practical reality of the principles. Fourth, there are unresolved tensions between some of the broad concepts themselves, particularly in many of the situations encountered by social care agencies. What happens when respect for someone leads workers to overrule her or his autonomy in the interests of longer-term survival and 'personhood'? What should be done when one person is harming another, or where competing interests collide (Horne 1987)? The problem here is that the strong humanist tradition from which this value base derives assumes that common natural capacities, needs and wants can be developed by rational guidance (Rojek *et al.* 1988), that there will be consensus about what is right, and that the key to self-actualization is in the hands of the individual. This leads to the fifth concern, the danger that when every individual is seen as unique and self-determining, collective need experienced by groups of people is overlooked, and the barriers to 'fulfilment' experienced as a result of structural inequality are ignored. If everyone is unique, everyone is, in effect, the same, and provided equal access is offered to the same facilities, people are being fair; or are they? Society's resources are unequally shared, and self-determination for a black elder who has no state pension, no housing rights, language barriers and is on a hospital waiting list for specialist health care will be very different from that for a retired, white, self-employed owner-occupier with a private health care scheme.

Paternalism and protection

Service users, in the picture of social care provision painted by policy guidance, are voluntary recipients of services, involved with agencies because they 'choose' to be. Within the rational consensus model, people who run risks because of frailty or vulnerability of some kind, or who pose risks to others, will be happy to receive a level of service commensurate with that which is necessary to afford an appropriate degree of protection against those risks. In reality, of course, this is not always the case. Some people will disagree about the risks they run to their own well-being or pose to that of others. Some people will recognize the risks but reject the services or provision offered. The traditional value system is ready for such eventualities. While generally preferring to promote autonomy, self-determination and choice, a subset of values proposes that it is sometimes right to depart from these if circumstances require it. Confidentiality, for instance, 'may be breached where it is demonstrably in the client's interests or where there is an overriding concern for the rights of other people, when for example the behaviour of the client may endanger others' (Social Care Association 1988).

The presence of certain 'conditions', such as learning disability or a mental health problem, often increases the likelihood that intervention in someone's best interests, or for his or her protection, will be made by those trusted to know best, a power sometimes vested in professionals. The Mental Health Act 1983, for example, allows the compulsory detention in hospital of someone with a mental disorder provided the disorder is of a nature or degree to warrant such detention and that detention is necessary in the interests of her or his own health or safety, or for the protection of others. In certain circumstances psychiatric treatment may be administered to compulsorily detained patients without their consent.

People with learning disability, if unable to consent to medical treatment, may be treated provided it is in their best interests and is in line with an accepted body of medical opinion. Thus the law reflects societal acceptance of the view that protection from harm, or promotion of someone's health interests, is a value which can take precedence over autonomy of decision-making, choice and self-determination. In social care the final decision about what is in line with a user's best interests lies not with that person but with the professionals involved.

The principles of 'best interests' and 'protection' are challenged primarily from the self-advocacy movement, particularly in the field of mental health, where opinion about the Mental Health Act 1983 is wide-ranging. Some people argue that denying civil liberties on the predictive opinion of professionals is an act of oppression and abuse *per se* (Chamberlin 1988; Plumb 1993). Other objections are raised on the grounds that 'protective' powers are liable to be abused by dominant groups as thinly disguised tools of social control (Fernando 1991; Ussher 1991). Others dispute the 'best interests' evidence, pointing to the inappropriate and damaging effects of provision that is intended to be therapeutic (Women in Mind 1986; Good Practices in Mental Health (GPMH) 1988; Johnstone 1989) and pointing the way to alternative definitions of how workers might best serve the interests of people in distress (Brandon 1991a). At the other end of the spectrum is the view that mental disorder justifies making decisions on behalf of other people, and that workers should be more prepared, not less, to intervene in the best interests of someone whose judgement is 'temporarily impaired'. Clearly there are variable and competing definitions and interpretations of 'best interests', along with a wide range of views on how 'protection' might best be offered, indicating that, in this field of values too, consensus is far from established.

Normalization

Normalization as a core value in social care has achieved widespread application in relation to services for people with disabilities. It is broadly understood as 'the principle by which people with a disability have the right to lead a valued ordinary life, based on the belief in their equality as human beings and citizens' (Ramon 1991b). It 'starts from the premise that a major handicap of disabled people is their devaluation in society, and it seeks to remedy this by enabling disabled people, as far as possible, to have experiences that are generally valued in society' (Wolfensberger 1972). Service models that group people together artificially by reference to perceived impairment contribute to negative social role attribution and labelling, which then compounds the process of devaluation, segregation and stigma. Services, therefore, must aim 'to promote patterns of life and conditions of everyday living which are as close as possible to the regular circumstances and ways of society' (Ryan and Thomas 1993).

During the 1980s service planning and design were greatly influenced by two associated principles derived from the concept of normalization. *Ordinary life* principles (Kings Fund 1983) prioritized ordinary housing and the delivery of services based on individual need 'to support community membership'. *Social role valorization* as a principle sought to enhance the perceived status of people with disabilities through their performance of socially desired and valued roles (Ramon 1991b). 'The most explicit and highest goal of normalisation must be the creation, support and defence of valued social roles for people who are at risk of social devaluation' (Wolfensberger 1983). Such a process has three major components (Baxter *et al.* 1990):

* to enable people to lead normal and valued lives;
* to do this by valued means, using services which are used by the whole community;
* to change attitudes so that people with disabilities are respected and valued.

Institutional living is seen as anathema to ordinary life, but there is also concern to ensure that the features of institutions, the loss of dignity, privacy, choice and control, are not merely translated into community care (Ramon 1991b). Opportunities for ordinary living must extend across all the major areas of valued activity: housing, income, health, education, and social, emotional and sexual relationships.

O'Brien (1986) proposes five 'accomplishments' that service users should be empowered by services to achieve:

* community presence – people have the right to experience a wide range of ordinary activities in the community, not in segregated provision;
* community participation – people have a right to engage in a wide range of relationships, with a wide range of people;

- choice – services must maximize opportunities for choice, making use of information and advocacy initiatives;
- competence – people must have opportunities to develop their strengths, skills and interests in ways that are functional and meaningful in the context of the ordinary community environments they occupy;
- respect – services must work to enhance the reputation of users and contribute to promoting their citizenship through presenting positive images.

To this must be added partnership (SSI 1993b) – the process of working together to enhance both the level of participation and the degree of control experienced by people in their relationship with service providers.

The broad themes within this value base can be identified: integration rather than segregation of people; promoting their rights and strengths rather than focusing on their risks; independence rather than dependency; developing skills and abilities rather than maintaining known competencies; fostering autonomy rather than paternalism and protection.

Normalization principles, however, despite their widespread influence have not avoided criticism. Within such a broad concept, there is infinite room for variation, and evidence exists that the interpretation of the principles is widely variable in terms of their impact on the nature and pattern of services (Allen *et al.* 1992). Claims to 'normality' often adopt an unquestioning view of what it is. As a consequence (Ryan and Thomas 1993):

- people with disabilities have conventional and conformist lifestyles imposed upon them, replicating the inequalities and divisions arising, for example, from stereotypical gender roles within families, or from the assumed normality of heterosexuality;
- people experience pressure to adjust to prevailing customs and standards, to make a better adjustment to society, rather than a focus on society's need to change to accommodate them;
- little attention is given to the structures needed to support people's right to ordinary housing and work, or to the barriers that have to be removed before such facilities are truly accessible.

Often what is seen as 'normal' or 'socially valued' is a majority-led definition (Ramon 1991b) which encompasses entrenched social values and beliefs that are not universal, and which fail to take account of the norms and patterns of black and minority ethnic communities. Some of the management and planning systems designed to enhance the implementation of normalization, such as PASS (Program Analysis of Service Systems) and IPP (Individual Programme Planning), are open to criticism because they apply white European norms and rely on cultural stereotyping (Baxter *et al.* 1990).

Finally, the processes of negative labelling and stigma are deeply ingrained within society, and highly resistant to change, with the result that 'the community' sometimes offers very limited opportunities for contact, integration, tolerance and acceptance (Day 1987), such that for some individuals persistent, negative feedback is an integral part of their experience, weakening and minimizing the benefits of normalization.

Equal opportunities and anti-discriminatory practice

'A social care worker shall not discriminate against any client on the grounds of race, nationality, sex, age, beliefs, sexual orientation or social standing, and shall work . . . to give equal opportunity for each client to achieve the maximum benefit and potential consistent with respecting the dignity and value of fellow human beings' (Social Care Association 1988).

This is not untypical of the broad catch-all statements which have become standard items since the mid-1980s in codes of practice and agency policy statements. Such statements represent a response to mounting evidence of how inequality arising from structural divisions in society is reflected in social care provision. Thus services are dominated by norms, standards and expectations set by more powerful groups in society, by white people rather than black, by men rather than women, non-disabled rather than disabled people, heterosexual people rather than gay men and lesbians, of an age range associated with economic productivity rather than younger or older people, rich rather than poor. The dominant norms are imbued with stereo-typical assumptions about those who are 'different' from the norm: that black families do not need services because 'they look after each other'; that it is legitimate to construct services around the caring family role of women; that physical impairment or mental disability entails dependency; that old age is a period of withdrawal and social decline; that people are poor because they have used their resources irresponsibly; that gay men and lesbian couples are unnatural and do not have the same partnership rights and needs as heterosexuals.

Using such stereotypes to justify bias and inequality in service provision has been increasingly challenged, and while concern for social justice takes a broad perspective and recognizes a wide range of sources of inequality, there has been particular emphasis on the widespread and enduring discrimi-nation experienced by black people. Social services departments, for instance, are seen as predominantly white organizations, catering for the needs of white people (A. Ahmad 1990). Black people are consistently under-represented as consumers of beneficial and supportive social care services, while they are over-represented as recipients of the more controlling aspects of social care, such as compulsory admission to psychiatric hospital (Barnes et al. 1990; Fernando 1991).

Within this context, equal opportunities and anti-discriminatory practice have specific meanings and emphases. An equal opportunities approach focuses on ensuring that barriers to accessing existing services are removed. Information is prioritized, and disseminated in formats accessible to and through locations used by the groups of people who are under-represented, to ensure they know what is available. There are attempts to ensure that decision-making is fair, that criteria on eligibility for services are applied equitably, without stereotypical assumptions about, for example, the cap-abilities of men and women in undertaking domestic tasks. Such a focus will often be combined with an emphasis on equal opportunities in the workplace: recruitment and selection procedures designed to encourage more black ap-plicants, increase numbers of disabled people in the workplace and promote more women into management; assurance to employees that they will not be discriminated against on grounds of sexuality; proactive policies to help carers to balance the demands of work and domestic care tasks.

Anti-discriminatory practice goes a step further in its recognition that the barriers to service use may reside in the services themselves, so that existing services will need to be reviewed to identify disincentives to their use (for example, day care activities dominated by cultural norms alien to some potential users, or inappropriate dietary provision which does not take account of religious requirements) and to develop more ethnically sensitive or gender appropriate services.

The equal opportunities and anti-discriminatory value base operates at both personal and organizational levels. Practitioners will have a commitment to examining their own attitudes and assumptions about people who are different from themselves, to identify and avoid the bias, stereotyping and prejudice that lead to discrimination. Agencies will commonly engage in the rhetoric of policy and position statements expressing the intention that people should have equality of opportunity in their use of services and laying a responsibility on staff not to discriminate in their work.

Such principles and commitments are clearly important but they are incomplete. Equal opportunity policy statements rarely result in the kind of detailed planning of the strategic steps and practical actions necessary to turn rhetoric into reality. If people are serious about tackling discrimination, a systematic framework must be established to achieve this, both organizationally and at an individual level (A. Ahmad 1990). Moreover, the emphasis in equal opportunities and anti-discriminatory practice is on voluntarism, people changing their practice because they want to, because they believe it is the right thing to do. Evidence indicates that reliance on this motivation is insufficient and that more effective and rapid change is achieved when rewards and sanctions are combined in an appropriate balance (Smockum 1991). The absence of effective anti-discriminatory legislation is material here. There is still no legal protection against discrimination on grounds of disability, mental health, sexuality, age and religion. Even legislation that does exist is largely ineffective. The Disabled Persons Employment Acts (1944, 1958) are honoured more in breach than observance (Janner 1990), with no effective sanction being imposed on employers who ignore the requirement to employ people with disabilities. Section 71 of the Race Relations Act 1976, which requires local authorities to ensure that their functions are performed with due regard to the need to eliminate unlawful discrimination and to promote equality of opportunity and good relations between people of different racial groups, is widely ignored and rarely used to back the necessary changes to policy and practice. Redress for discrimination on grounds of either race or sex (RRA 1976, SDA 1975) is still dependent upon an individual complainant being prepared to pursue her or his case and, even where a challenge is forthcoming, evidence for discrimination is exceedingly difficult to find.

Another problem with this value base is its assumption that remedial action is sufficient: that removing barriers and creating equality of opportunity will of itself create equality of outcome; that action by individual practitioners can be decisive in changing a service user's experience. These things are important, but to rely solely upon them ignores how inequality is endemic to the whole fabric of society, how widespread and pervasive structural oppression shapes and determines people's experience in a way which requires structural change to achieve significant impact. People who use social care services may have experienced longstanding discrimination in education, health care, housing and employment; they may have experienced racism, gender oppression, segregation and isolation from the mainstream of society, deprivation of their civil liberty and attacks on their citizenship status. Thus, while personal and organizational action for equality is important, its focus must be wider than merely the relationship created through use of services if equality is to be addressed on a significant scale.

Partnership

Partnership between service users and providers is promoted in government guidance as a key foundation of community care services, appearing in association with words such as consultation, choice and user involvement. Partnership is also a key concept in the professional value base underpinning community care: the word appears consistently in professional literature, agency policy documents and practitioner parlance. With the common themes of showing greater respect for service users' views and increasing their say in the development and delivery of services (Newton and Marsh 1993), it is a process where the key stakeholders in a service, especially provider and user, cooperate in defining how the service should be designed and delivered (Newman 1993). It attempts to clarify and sometimes to alter the balance of power within the relationship.

There have been attempts to clarify the principles upon which partnership practice is based. Marsh and Fisher (1992) propose that:

- the investigation of problems must be with the explicit consent of the potential user, or must be the minimum necessary to be consistent with statutory duties;
- user agreement, or a clear statutory mandate, must be the basis of intervention;
- intervention must be based on the views of all relevant family members and carers;
- services must be based on negotiated agreement and not on assumptions or prejudices about users' behaviour and wishes;
- users must have the greatest possible choice in the services they are offered.

Key objectives within such a model will be (Braye and Preston-Shoot 1993a):

- open dialogue with service users such that their views and concerns are represented in problem definition, in prioritization of needs to be addressed and in decision-making;
- clear definition of aims and the setting of achievable goals;
- honesty about differences of opinion and how they are affected by the power held by the different parties in the partnership;

- user access to information to promote informed understanding and consent, and to complaints procedures to promote accountability.

Partnership is promoted at several levels. In the context of an individual's use of social care services, the principle requires an open process of negotiation about needs, the means of meeting them, the level and form of service provision. In an organizational context, it requires an openness to consultation and feedback about services, and user involvement in planning for development.

The apparent consensus about partnership as an uncontroversial 'good thing' masks what is in fact a complex and varied aetiology in which several influential factors are combined (Braye and Preston-Shoot 1992b).

- Consumerism in the market place: the belief that economy, efficiency and effectiveness in social care provision will best be served by 'consumers' of services having choice between diverse forms of provision, and regulating its quality by exercising their 'purchasing power', which requires providers and enablers of services to be responsive to consumer demands. In this system, partnership is required in order to get close enough to consumers to understand their demands and requirements.
- Individual and family autonomy and responsibility: the individual consumerist ideology is founded on the belief that individuals are self-determining and ultimately responsible for themselves and for those within their family network. Thus state intervention is neither a given nor a right; nor should the state impose – the relationship is one to be negotiated – a partnership in which both have responsibilities. The state may provide to promote, but not to take over, the function of self and family responsibility.
- The curtailment of professional power: this arises from two quite different directions. First, social care professions, especially social work, have moved to challenge their own power base, both in questioning the assumed right of those with professional status to impose their opinions on people's lives and in identifying their contribution to discrimination. Within this context partnership becomes a professional requirement, a vehicle for collaboration which values and respects the views and rights of those who use services, and a means of working with people to promote their interests. Second, there is the impetus to make professionals more accountable, not to those who use their services but to the state which regulates their powers and duties. Unfettered professional discretion that is outside political control can be inconvenient. A requirement to work in partnership, particularly when the interests so promoted will be many and varied, brings a series of checks and balances to professional autonomy and power.
- The emergence of a strong self-advocacy movement: it would be misleading to allow the credit for partnership to be taken by dominant and powerful groups in society, as if it happens solely because they allow and encourage it. The influence of self-advocacy must be acknowledged – people who use services speaking out *against* the imposition of professional decisions 'in their best interests' and *for* a stronger voice in decisions affecting their lives. The irony is that self-advocacy demands more than

involvement in decision-making and consultation about services. It emerges from the politics of liberation (Beresford and Croft 1990) and demands real power to *affect* decision-making, emancipation not paternalism. Partnership here is a professional-led response to these demands, one which attempts still to work within existing power relationships and traditional definitions. 'Only the poor are offered partnership – the rest of us usually prefer to control the services we receive, or pay others to do the job for us' (Newman 1993).

The complexity of the background to partnership, and the competing interests residing therein, make it difficult for partnership to achieve a practice reality. A wide gap exists between intention and implementation (Marsh and Fisher 1992). The reasons why the thought does not guarantee the deed will be explored further in Chapter 5.

Radical values

There is a more radical agenda than any of the preceding attempts to reform the relationship between service providers and users. The reformist agenda builds essentially on key assumptions: that inequalities are an inevitable feature of social organization; that a caring society will provide for those unable through incapacity to improve their lot, and should do so in as humane a way as possible; that individuals, given equal opportunity, have within themselves the potential to remove barriers to personal success and are themselves responsible for doing so. The professional value base informs the task of ameliorating conditions within that system, but without changing its inherent form or structure.

The radical value base starts from a different premise: that an individual's life chances are determined by her or his position in society's structure, a structure characterized by social division along lines of race, class and gender, which organizes further major differentiation along criteria such as age, (dis)ability, sexuality, health status, religion, ethnic origin and cultural practices. Inequality exists in the relative power held by such groupings to gain and sustain valued commodities and advantages. Being white, male, non-disabled, of an age to contribute to economic productivity, brings more power than being black, female, disabled, old or very young. Individual need or suffering is thus part of a collective experience shared by a group of people, and must be addressed through collective action. To do otherwise is to mask the need for structural change and reduce its likelihood (Bamford 1989).

Essential to this analysis are the concepts of *power* and *oppression* (Ward and Mullender 1991). Where relations are so structured that one person or group of people benefits at the expense of another person or group, then the people who benefit have greater power in those relations. The power can be manifest at an individual, family, group, community or societal level, and can take material and emotional forms (McNay 1992). Powerful groups not only have the *power to* (to do, to achieve, to exercise choice, to influence), they also have *power over* (over others, to coerce and inflict their authority) (Hugman 1991), through control of social institutions which can be manipulated to maintain their interests. This exploitation and denial of the interests of less powerful groups constitutes oppression, which is the process by which individuals or groups with ascribed or achieved power unjustly limit the lives, experiences and/or opportunities of those with less power (NCVS 1989). Such a perspective entails a distinctly different view of values, moving them from their position as a discrete personal statement to part of an ideological perspective on the socio-economic system (Bamford 1989). The growing recognition during the 1980s of the impact of oppression on the lives of people using social care services led to the development of an alternative value base which:

• recognizes the socio-political context of service users' life experiences, and of the agency's role and function in that context;
• aims to ensure that the ways in which services are provided do not contribute to oppression;
• aims to assist users in their struggles against oppression (Thompson 1993).

Various processes have contributed to an understanding of how power and oppression affect people who use social care services. The first has been a process of isolating a single dimension of experience, such as being black, female or working class, and throwing it into sharp relief in order to understand the power dynamics involved and their impact upon those oppressed by virtue of their belonging to that single group. Thus an understanding has developed of Britain as a white dominated society in which racism is endemic, fed by a historical view of black people as inferior, in itself a stereotype constructed to justify economic and social exploitation. 'Racism is recognised not just as a personal prejudice but as an institutional phenomenon which occurs when individuals, in carrying out routine practices of their employment or institution, produce outcomes which in their effect discriminate against members of ethnic minority populations' (Husband 1991). The professional value base has thus developed an anti-racist agenda committed to combating racism not only within personal professional practice but also on the wider institutional front (CCETSW 1991a).

Feminist critiques have similarly developed an understanding of how patriarchal power relations shape women's experience in all spheres from the private family domain through to public life (Langan 1992). A recognition of the inequality and oppression experienced by women has had an impact on social policy and social care, particularly social work (Hudson *et al.* 1993), and has contributed to a prioritization of gender awareness in the professional value base (Hanmer and Statham 1988; Dominelli and McLeod 1989; Phillipson 1992).

Disability is a further dimension of experience that has been singled out, with a focus on the oppression experienced through the imposition of devaluing and segregated services, through exclusion from the facilities and social benefits enjoyed by other citizens, and through institutional discrimination which both denies disabled people their chosen lifestyles and colludes with unequal treatment and outcomes in areas such as housing, income and employment (Oliver and Barnes 1993). Understanding how an individual's experience of disability is created in interactions with a physical and social world designed for non-disabled living (Swain *et al.* 1993), and recognizing the assumptions that inform dominant orthodoxy about the identity and ability of disabled people (Barton 1993), lead to a value position which sees disability as a human rights issue requiring political action rather than a social problem requiring welfare provision (Oliver 1991/2).

Further single dimensions have been identified and explored: oppression arising through ageism, the social process through which negative images of and attitudes towards older people, based on stereotyping old age as a period of decline and dependence, result in discrimination (Hughes and Mtezuka 1992); the impact of homophobia and heterosexism, resulting in either unrecognized and ignored needs or negative and controlling responses (Brown 1992); the exclusion and abuse of people with mental health problems (Rogers et al. 1993), both in the name of treatment 'in their best interests' and as a result of fear, labelling and stigma in society.

The second process, following from that of broad differentiation along one dimension, has been recognition of further differentiation and complexity according to each individual's experience of oppression. This has entailed awareness of the diversities between people in the same oppressed group, recognition that 'none of us belongs to one social compartment' and that attempts to reduce the complexities of people's experience to neat little boxes labelled 'race', 'gender' and 'class' (Hudson *et al.* 1993) result in simplistic responses.

Feminism, in its prioritization of women's oppression, failed to find a role in the picture for older women, colluding with ageist stereotypes of older people as a burden on younger women (Hughes and Mtezuka 1992). The avoidance by the disability movement of a focus on the personal experience of disability, within an understanding of the social oppression arising from disability, can be seen as a consequence of the disability movement's domination by men (Morris 1991). Women's analyses have demonstrated how the social construct of gender plays an important part in the lives of disabled women *and* men (Lonsdale 1990; Lloyd 1992; Morris 1993c). The impact of race, of being black and a woman, black and disabled, has been ignored by an assumption within the dominant single oppression model of white European culture as a benchmark, to the extent that black people are often invisible within broad groupings (Francis 1993). Attempts to recognize the multiple and variable impacts of differing forms of oppression led to concepts such as 'double oppression' to reflect the experience of being black and gay, or 'triple oppression' in the case of someone who was, additionally, disabled or in old age, as if it were simply a question of multiplying the factors to reach an understanding of 'how oppressed' an individual might be. This notion has been rejected as under-estimating how forms of oppression interact to create a unique experience. It has been replaced by a preference for the concept of 'simultaneous oppression' – a distinct and separate experience and identity which can result in an individual being separate from and marginalized by *all* groups to which she or he might belong (Stuart 1993). Thus a radical value base, in attempting to account for and respond to such processes, has moved to an integrated model which recognizes the complexity and diversity of the manifold oppressions that affect people's lives (Langan 1992).

In essence, radical values espouse social change goals, taking seriously the responsibility to engage with and speak out in the debate about welfare in the light of mounting evidence of inequalities, injustice, poverty and despair (Jones 1993). The implications for the direction of social care practice are profound. At the heart of practice informed by this value base is the concept of *empowerment*. This is valued both as an end in itself and as a means of achieving social change (Stevenson and Parsloe 1993). In this context empowerment is very different from its promotion in community care guidance. There it becomes the essential expression of individualism under New Right welfare consumerism. Here it gives expression to the collective voice of universal need (Ward and Mullender 1991) and derives its substance and focus from a user movement demanding control. Control is a common theme of definitions. Empowerment means:

- extending one's ability to take effective decisions (Meade and Carter 1990);
- individuals, groups and/or communities taking control of their circumstances and achieving their own goals, thereby being able to work towards maximizing the quality of their lives (Adams 1990);
- enabling people who are disempowered to have more control over their lives, to have a greater voice in institutions, services and situations which affect them, and to exercise power over someone else rather than simply being recipients of exercised power (Croft and Beresford 1993);
- helping people to regain their own power (Read and Wallcraft, 1992).

The value of empowerment finds expression in several approaches to practice. There is a concern to ensure that service provision does not in itself oppress. 'The personal powerlessness experienced by those undergoing mental distress is compounded by a service which denies choice and dignity and is underpinned by the threat of compulsion' (Barker 1991). Services will value and build on people's strengths rather than focus on their deficits, and will attempt to tap into the strength developed in enduring oppression, both as a source of personal power and as a contribution to collective strength derived through meeting together and developing shared agendas (Barker and Peck 1987). This may involve separatist provision: women only, black groups, lesbian or gay collectives, organizations of disabled people. Collective endeavour has led to the development of a strong and active user movement in several social care fields. The mental health survivors' movement, for example, developed nationally from individual groups in different parts of Britain meeting and inspiring each other (Beeforth *et al.* 1990), and has produced common themes which find echoes in both organizations of disabled people and the users of learning disability services:

- that users have the right and the ability to be involved in the planning, management and delivery of services in both statutory agencies and their own organizations;
- that users gain power from working in groups;
- that service planners and providers must recognize and give status and resources to users (Thompson 1991).

Self-advocacy has, however, a wider agenda of improving not just service provision but also the status of service recipients in society (Campbell 1990). People in effect want more say in their lives, not just in services (Beresford 1993), and the goals of change within an empowerment value base will extend beyond the service provision agenda to wider avenues of citizenship in which oppression, whatever its source, is experienced. The content of the agenda remains essentially for service users to define; it is the process which is defined by the value base, summarized by Mullender and Ward (1991) as:

- all people have skills, understanding and ability;
- people have rights to be heard, to participate, to choose, to define problems and action;
- people's problems are complex and social oppression is a contributory factor;
- people acting collectively are powerful;
- methods of work must be non-elitist and non-oppressive.

In the two broad categories of values identified as influential in social care practice, tensions are obvious between the radical and the traditional agendas, between an approach which makes issues out of cases and one which makes cases out of issues (Howe 1979). These tensions surface in statements about the competencies required of qualified social workers. They must respect established traditional rights such as dignity, privacy, confidentiality and choice; yet they must understand and counteract discrimination, demonstrate anti-racist and anti-sexist practice, and seek to promote policies that are anti-oppressive and anti-discriminatory (CCETSW 1991b). This is tantamount to saying that power and privilege must be challenged but without upsetting the legal and moral foundations of economic and political individualism on which they are built (Jordan 1991). The tension is compounded by criticisms that may be made of each from the perspective of the other. Professionals can be seen as upholding a system of distribution of opportunity that is profoundly unequal by focusing on individuals rather than on structures (Wilding 1982). Conversely, a focus on the individual user–professional relationship can be seen as primary and essential to personal well-being and development (Onyett 1992). Certainly the traditional agenda and its emphasis on the individual is more familiar territory for social care professionals. An analysis of a variety of agencies' value statements, position statements and declarations of principle and intent (Bornat 1993) reveals common demands for recognition of the unique nature of individual need, for human rights, liberty, privacy, normalization and equality of opportunity. Participation, consultation and representation, information and choice are frequently prioritized. What is often missing is the focus on collective action, and the wider challenge to oppression in arenas other than the delivery of services.

Further complications arise from the use of the same terminology to signify widely varying concepts. The terms participation, involvement and partnership are used interchangeably without differentiation (Barker and Peck 1987), yet mean widely differing things to different groups of people, and can reflect both consumerist and democratic agendas (Beresford and Croft

1993). The term 'anti-discriminatory practice' similarly holds widely differing meanings: from 'treating people as individuals' to 'treating people equally'; from 'being about race, class and gender' to 'not just being about race, class and gender' (Balen *et al.* 1993). 'Empowerment' itself, welcomed in all quarters as a 'good thing', can change its meaning (Gomm 1993). In the radical value base it involves working alongside oppressed people to challenge the source of their oppression in the abuse of power by others. Borrowed by the traditional value base it is used to describe a process of enabling people to acquire the skills and self-confidence needed to bring about improvements in the quality of their lives, or helping people to compete more effectively for scarce resources. In both it can involve a process of cutting professionals down to size, and making them more responsive and accountable to people who use their services. A danger exists that one meaning masquerades as another, leading to a process whereby use of the term to describe professionally led initiatives acts as a 'social aerosol', covering up the disturbing smell of conflict and division (Mullender and Ward 1991).

Initiatives which appear to stem from a particular value base can in fact have widely differing aims. Service user involvement, for example, does not necessarily lead to empowerment. Within a consumerist agenda it becomes a means of gaining information to preserve a market position, a means of targeting need more efficiently but without any change to the power balance in decision-making or control of services (Croft and Beresford 1993). Involvement even with the goal of empowerment can, additionally, reflect the sometimes competing perspectives of parties with a legitimate interest. Debates around the impact of community care policy, with its emphasis on informal care networks, provide a good example of the complex interplay between the interests thus identified: those of a disability movement which advocates not for care and carers but for resources to control; those of carers wanting recognition and support; and those of feminist challenges to the concept of family care on the grounds of its exploitation of women (Parker 1993).

The complications and complexities of power and empowerment in the context of social care practice will be further explored in Chapter 5.

Insofar as the value base for practice is concerned, it is important to recognize and understand the factors which impact upon the development of a particular set of values and upon the choices that are available to workers and users when they prioritize certain values in certain situations. There are several influential factors here:

- models used to assist understanding of the experiences and needs which bring people to social care agencies;
- the organizational context in which social care practice occurs;
- the personal history and experiences that workers bring to their practice.

Models for understanding

The experiences and needs which bring people into contact with social care agencies, be they related to age, physical impairment, learning disability or mental health problems, have in common that they can be understood and explained by reference to a number of different 'causative' factors:

- factors pertaining to the individual and her or his internal processes, i.e. physical ageing, a medical condition, a genetic factor, physical damage;
- factors associated with the individual in his or her immediate environment – relationships, occupation, stress levels – and the interaction between them;
- factors associated with the individual in the context of social groupings, and her or his position within society's structure.

Implicit throughout government policy on community care is an assumption that people's needs arise because of the inevitable frailty of older age, because of physical incapacity to perform self-care tasks, because of mental incapacity to make sound and safe decisions or to heed risks and danger. Physical disability, for example, is seen as arising from a clinical condition, a disease process, illness, genetic disorder or functional bodily impairment, with 'treatment' geared to replacing the missing function and/or minimizing the effects of the impairment. Thus care is provided to do things *for* people that they are prevented from doing for themselves. Special equipment is provided to assist them in adapting to the physical environment. In the context of this explanation, the disability is construed as a personal tragedy, characterized by an experience of loss for both the individual and those close to him or her, particularly in cases of acquired or progressive impairment. Part of the professional task is to assist with the psychological and emotional adjustment of 'coming to terms' with the disability and its effects, to help people to adapt to the changes of functional ability and relationships that are entailed and to resolve their feelings about lost or never to be experienced opportunities.

Similarly, medical explanations, oriented towards the individual and his or her immediate social context, are also apparent in the mental health field. Mental 'disorders' such as schizophrenia or severe depression are deemed to arise from the presence of genetic or biological factors, from identifiable biochemical processes, and to be treatable by pharmacological intervention once recognized and correctly diagnosed. Alternative causative theories focus on the impact of immediate environmental factors that are deemed to be stressful and damaging to emotional well-being – experiences of loss and bereavement, of stressful relationships or living conditions. Intervention here focuses on psychosocial approaches – counselling, small-scale environmental adjustment, work on relationships and coping strategies.

Such services in the mental health and disability fields are constructed around a view of individuals having personal problems arising from some kind of functional deficit (Finkelstein 1993a), whether that be in physical incapacity or emotional vulnerability. The response is to cure or to care, to create an enforced dependency, requiring need to be medicalized and individualized in order to gain provision of a basic service (Morris 1993d) and the service to be packaged in the context of some kind of therapeutic casework relationship (Barber 1991). These 'explanations' are accompanied by negative stereotyping which both contributes to and justifies the service response: disabled people as brave, tragic, hopeless or useless; people with mental health problems as self-destructive or dangerous to others. Such images are widespread and in common public currency (Spastics Society 1991).

Similar processes are observable in older people's services, where negative assumptions about older age as 'decline' and a burden lead to low expectations, both of the services and of individuals themselves. At its most negative the consequences of enduring any such condition or impairment have been seen as tantamount to 'social death', an inevitable withdrawal and marginalization from the mainstream of society, with the professional role focused on managing the time-space between social and actual death (Finkelstein 1991).

The alternatives to these very individualized explanations of people's needs and experiences may be termed structural explanations, which locate the experience of disability or of mental health problems or of older age within its social context, taking account of how that context is created by social structures, norms and expectations. The disabled people's movement proposes a model for understanding disability in which it is seen to stem from the failure of the social environment to adjust to the needs and aspirations of citizens with disabilities (Barton 1993). The turning point in this thinking occurred in response to the social death model of disability in the 1970s (Finkelstein 1991) in the declaration from the Union of the Physically Impaired Against Segregation (UPIAS 1976) that disability is 'the disadvantage or restriction of activity caused by a contemporary social organisation which takes no or little account of people who have physical impairments and thus excludes them from participation in the mainstream of social activities. Physical disability is therefore a particular form of social oppression.' From such a perspective the service response must be to work with disabled people for the removal of the barriers experienced by them in a social world that is organized for able-bodiedness. The focus in such a model is on basic universal needs which are collectively voiced by organizations *of* disabled people – information, counselling, housing, technical assistance, personal assistance, transport and access (Davis 1991) – and on campaigning to stop the patronage which trades on negative images of disabled people used by charities such as Children in Need to raise money for things that should be a right (Morris 1991).

Similar alternatives to individualized medical or psychosocial models are available in the mental health context. 'Diagnosis is a neat way of creating order out of chaos, but cannot represent the experience of the user' (Onyett 1992). Social models of mental health offer a range of explanations: that emotional distress is the consequence of heightened sensitivity to the observed abuses of society, or a valid protest against powerlessness and oppression; more radically, that psychiatry holds a political function, serving the interests of the powerful by dealing with the problems created by an exploitative society, or exercising a form of social control, regulating 'abnormal', deviant or inconvenient behaviour by constructing it as 'illness'. Such explanations recognize that mental health problems have a social, environmental and political meaning (Onyett 1992), and propose that emotional distress thus needs a holistic, not a medical, approach (Read and Wallcraft 1992).

In both the disability and mental health fields the self-advocacy movement has been instrumental in promoting ways of understanding experiences and needs that move beyond individual pathology. While there are differences and subtleties of interpretation, there are commonalities and areas of solidarity which are emphasized. Key objectives are integration into the mainstream of society, a say in the provision of support services and securing the civil rights of citizenship (Beresford 1993), objectives echoed by the principles espoused by the independent living movement (Morris 1993d):

- all human life is of value;
- anyone, irrespective of impairment, is capable of exercising choice;
- people disabled by society's reaction to physical, intellectual and sensory impairment, and to emotional distress, have the right to assert control over their lives, and to participate fully in society.

The links between models for understanding the needs of people who use services and the value base underpinning practice are important to make. If a mental health problem is construed as resulting from disease processes that are treatable, workers may well decide that it is unethical to allow this unnecessary health risk to persist (Fisher *et al.* 1984) and thus be attracted to the value position that it is valid to intervene in people's best interests to protect them from the worst consequences of exercising their autonomy by refusing treatment. If a person's disability is defined as arising from exclusion from facilities rather than from functional impairment, workers' efforts will focus on changing the environment to remove the barriers, or providing resources to facilitate access, rather than upon providing individualized services which compound isolation. Workers' models of thinking encourage them towards a particular conceptualization of their professional task and will cause them to prioritize certain values over others.

The importance of these connections is increasingly being recognized, with recommendations that the models for understanding that are being used to inform policy and practice should be made explicit (SSI 1993b), and that 'to change practice it is necessary to change the assumptions people make about the individual and their [*sic*] problems and social problems' (Smale *et al.* 1993).

The organizational context

The organizational context for social care practice is the second factor impacting on the potential and opportunity to prioritize particular sets of values. The Barclay Report (1982) identified that social care practice must 'act within the law, agency policies and professional values', but which are determinative when is not clarified. At one level the bureaucratic organization of agencies constrains and erodes professional values, replacing them with technical and procedural decision-making (Cornwell 1992/3). Thus practice is led by bureaucratic rather than professional imperatives (Adams 1990). Organizational inertia is a major obstacle to the implementation of value principles in practice: where professional staff can with ease identify and articulate the practices that *should* arise from such principles, they have more difficulty believing that such practices *could* be implemented in *their* work setting, and even where value-led practice is considered possible there is less observable evidence of its implementation (Booth *et al.* 1990), a gap attributable primarily to factors located within the organization's policies and priorities.

More fundamentally, values are limited by what society will tolerate and sanction via the mandates which govern agency function (Horne 1987) and by the assumed expert role of professionals within that function (Finkelstein 1993b). Self-determination will thus be constrained by factors such as the level of agency resources and the professional role as gatekeeper to those resources, by society's use of an agency to ensure individuals' conformity to its expectations, by the perceived authority of workers and by other subtle interpersonal processes (Whittington 1971). The worker's professional values are far from being absolute or determinative in this context, and must be balanced by the need to assess, define and mediate between sometimes opposing interests which impose limitations (Horne 1987).

The potential conflict between certain values and the agency and social contexts in which social care takes place is illustrated in the varied competencies for social work (CCETSW 1991b), in which practitioners must counteract discrimination and oppression, mobilize users' rights and promote choice, yet also understand and act within organizational and legal structures and functions, even though these may reflect and contribute to the oppressions experienced by users (Preston-Shoot 1992). Indeed, the swing away from state welfare to individualism, familialism, voluntarism and private enterprise pushes professional practice remorselessly towards practices of surveillance, monitoring and control, with relationships between service users and practitioners characterized by antagonism and mistrust, directly at variance with the values of empowerment (Jones and Novak 1993).

Thus, while value-led initiatives might make cosmetic changes to practice, 'in a deeper and more general sense fundamental value assumptions are unchanged because they reflect the power of the institutionalised role of a bureaucratised profession in a complex modern state' (Payne 1989).

The personal context

The third factor that influences the implementation of values in practice is each individual's personal history, the experiences and learning that have shaped her or his view of society and motivation to enter social care practice, and that provide the foundation upon which professional values are subsequently built. The formulation of a personal value system is a complex process, influenced not only by personal and family circumstances, but also by class, race and gender, and experiences arising from (dis)ability, sexuality, health status, age and other factors of difference and potential inequality. Each individual will have experiences of his or her own oppression, of colluding with and contributing to the oppression of others, of recognizing and working to change such processes.

Vital to social care practice is an understanding of the impact of personal experience, and an awareness of how it affects orientation within the professional value system, requiring workers to learn, unlearn or relearn, and leading them to prioritize certain values over others. The exercises that follow are designed to assist this process of exploration.

Exercise 2.1.   Think of the earliest time you remember being aware of someone whose racial origin was different from your own. What messages did you receive about your racial identity and other people's racial identity? What effect has this had on your personal relationships and outlook, and on your work? Ask yourself similar questions about class, gender and disability. Critically appraise your practice: in what ways do you reinforce existing power structures, stereotypes and assumptions in your work?

Exercise 2.2.   Think of your work base. How easy is it for disabled people to use or gain access to it? Are there any changes you would like to see? Think of your home and ask the same questions.

Exercise 2.3.   Think of someone you work with, his or her experiences and the needs he or she presents. How could the situation be explained? What influences have there been upon his or her current position? Are there *different* explanations? How might these different explanations affect how you and others view him or her, and the services offered?

Exercise 2.4.   Spend some time looking through magazines and watching television adverts for portrayals of older people. What are the dominant images presented? What is the racial origin of the people portrayed? Are there differences between how men and women are portrayed? What role is economic status, or health, playing in how they are presented? What messages are these images portraying? What value statements are behind them?

Exercise 2.5.   Imagine you have the power to construct a society in which you are able to make it as *difficult* as possible for people with mental health problems to live. Consider any measures you wish: housing, income, occupation, health care, education, leisure, family policy. You may make different rules for women and men, black people and white people, people with money, etc. Now imagine you can reverse this process and create a society in which people with mental health problems can live with ease. Consider the same arenas as before. Which of these was the most difficult? Which society most resembles the society in which we live?

Exercise 2.6.   Scan the newspapers for reports that involve some area of discrimination by one group or person against another. Identify the grounds on which discrimination is taking place (or perhaps being proposed). What are your views?

Towards a synthesis of values

In separating out the different strands of values in social care, our purpose has been to identify and understand rather than to attempt to create distinct categories. The reality of practice is that the influences will be mixed and integrated to create a synthesis reflecting choices and priorities relevant in any one given situation. Both traditional and radical values have contributions to make.

Respect for persons in a context of anti-oppressive practice retains what is valuable and important between service user and provider as a core component of their relationship, without ignoring the wider political realities of people's lives. Confidentiality, in a negotiated agreement about its limits and boundaries, is a key component of trust and respect. Every part of social care practice, from helping someone to take a bath to speaking out on someone's behalf in support of her or his rights, can be done in ways which diminish or enhance personal dignity. Maximizing choice, where choice is genuine and significant, enhances control and is a form of empowerment. Partnership within an anti-oppressive value base becomes an approach for tackling the structures of oppression and resourcing people to take action against powerlessness.

There will be times when action must be taken to protect individuals from the harmful effects of either their own actions or those of others, for within a value base that prioritizes empowerment there must be limits to power and its potential abuse in respect of others.

The usefulness of differing models for understanding is apparent within a synthesis. Taking models of disability as an example, there is recognition that at different times and for different individuals, medical attention and a focus on functional capacity can be important. This is not to detract from the argument that the social and physical environment must itself adapt to ensure that it meets the needs and rights of disabled people, but rather to recognize that many people's experience is of an *interaction* between their impairment and the environment, which requires a focus on this middle ground in which the interaction occurs (French 1993). A similar perspective is important in mental health work – the recognition that, while the impact of mental health problems is experienced at the individual level of distress, their development is essentially socially constructed and must be understood in that context (Braye and Varley 1992). At the point of interface between the personal and the political both individual and collective approaches are important to address 'individual internalised structures and engage in social action to secure social change' (Frosh 1987), and to bring people together to break down the isolation that compounds powerlessness, promoting individual change as a precursor to social change driven collectively (Barber 1991).

What is apparent from this exploration of values in social care is that there is a wide gap between the professional value base and the policy context, with its language of economy, value for money, service specifications and contracts. The value base in effect requires social care agencies to take a much wider view of their role than that envisaged in government community care guidance, and to engage with a more radical definition of need. This discussion will be taken forward in Chapter 4. At the level of individual practice the challenge to practitioners of responding appropriately to policy guidance and values mandates will be discussed further in Chapter 3.

3 Training and

staff development

Accompanying the development of community care has been the recognition of its implications for the job roles and skill development of staff working in social care. In its original influential report the Audit Commission (1986) outlined some of the differences between work in residential care and in community care facilities, maintaining that staff in the latter must be able to work alone, make decisions and adjust to fluctuating needs – demands requiring qualities of flexibility, judgement and adaptability. Subsequent policy documentation and practice guidance (for example, DoH 1989a, 1990a) refer to the training implications of what is contained within them, also recognizing the impact on individuals of change and uncertainty and their consequent support needs (DoH 1991a). Much of the feedback from demonstration and pilot projects concerns the development and support needs of staff making transitions to new job roles (Knapp *et al*. 1992; Robbins 1993).

The demands are experienced at managerial, professional and vocational levels in an organization. Provision of social care is labour intensive. Staff must be equipped with new skills and enabled to work in new ways (DoH 1989a, 1990a; SSI 1990a).

A significant recognition was the emphasis on the increasing importance of the contribution of vocational staff, in addition to the new skills required by professional staff for resource management and the estimate that large numbers of domiciliary and residential care staff might legitimately require access to a training and qualification structure. The training requirements of an unknown number of staff in the independent sector were also acknowledged.

The government had in 1988 introduced financial support for training targeted on specific staff groups: a Training Support Grant made to local authorities contingent upon their own financial contribution and upon strategic planning for the implementation of training plans. In 1991 this support programme was extended to staff groups working with all community care service users in addition to those working predominantly with older people, and to resource strategies intended to address the training needs in the voluntary and independent sectors (DoH 1990a).

Alongside recognition of the training implications of policy change and practice development has been a similar emphasis on the importance of training staff in the value base underpinning their work. This has been apparent in both professional and vocational training arenas. CCETSW (1991b) has emphasized the role of values learning in social work qualifying training, and has promoted anti-oppressive practice training generally and anti-racist training more specifically through a range of publications (CCETSW 1991a; Ahmad-Aziz *et al.* 1992; Phillipson 1992; Bano *et al.* 1993). A similar trend has been in the development of National Vocational Qualifications in Care. Originally based on a functional analysis of the tasks undertaken by direct care workers, this was subsequently revised to give greater prominence to both the values and the knowledge base informing how these tasks are performed.

Despite this welcome prioritization of training and staff development in social care, there appears to be an underlying assumption which contradicts the more overt emphasis on skills and qualifications. This is the tendency to downgrade and devalue direct care work to the status of 'routine tending' – an automatic, common-sense function that can be undertaken by anyone (Grimwood and Popplestone 1993) because it is an extension of domestic work (Douglas and Payne 1988) and comes naturally from 'the right people' (Staton 1993). The fact that direct care workers undertake tasks commonly also undertaken by unpaid family or volunteer carers makes direct care work susceptible to the traditional view that it is a vocation and somehow different in quality from other aspects of social care provision, and that it is done for love, duty or moral satisfaction rather than money or career advancement (Butler 1991). When seen in the context of gender role stereotyping, these assumptions both explain and compound the position of the predominantly female workforce in this social care sector. The 'professional' side of social care is seen as planning, negotiating, purchasing and financial management functions. The function of direct care provision is seen as vocational, requiring a vocational rather than professional qualification (DoH 1989a). This split is reflected in feedback about the training needs arising in demonstration projects – seen as needing to be a blend of therapeutic and basic skills, professional attitudes and caring (Knapp *et al.* 1992; Knapp 1993).

The devaluation of direct care provider skills is also apparent in the fact that, throughout the guidance documents on community care, where training is mentioned the emphasis is on training for the assessment, planning, care management and contract specification functions, in effect the management and *purchasing* of social care (Riches 1993). The training needs of providers have been relatively ignored (Bell 1993), with the assumption that skills reside in functions – that purchasers need assessment skills while providers need human relationship skills, whereas the reality is that not only are the functions artificially segregated but also workers representing both ends of the market need skills in common with each.

Factors influencing training strategies

Various factors contribute to the recognition that training and staff development strategies are important to the implementation of community care. Job roles are undergoing fundamental change because of the accelerated policy shift. This is apparent both within and between disciplines. The tradition of segregating and institutionalizing disabled people has meant that community-based workers are more accustomed to offering services to non-disabled people, and consequently have to extend both knowledge and skills, in addition perhaps to encountering challenges to values. Conversely, staff who have worked with disabled people have predominantly done so in segregated settings, and have to adapt to the differing demands of community-based care (Segal 1991). Evidence exists that care staff experience ambiguity when asked to perform as independent practitioners in the community, and that training has a key role in preventing a slide into low morale and high staff turnover (Robbins 1993). A needs-led service demands much of frontline staff, especially an unusual degree of flexibility. Without training and support this is likely to produce casualties (Knapp *et al.* 1992).

For other staff, community-based working entails a shift away from focusing on individual service users to working with community groups or supporting carers (Henderson and Armstrong 1993). The home care service is focusing less on domestic tasks and more on personal care (NUPE 1993), encroaching on community nursing roles which bring new training needs (Francis 1992). Similar processes of change are apparent in nursing where understandings about the social determinants of health have meant recognition of the need for a nursing model capable of responding to these, independently of medical intervention, and to potential overlaps with social care roles (Bywaters 1987). Thus major changes and developments in job roles in primary health care and reviews of the skill mix required (Risdale 1993) run parallel to the job role development processes in the social care world, the differences and overlap between them being made more significant by the shared care initiatives heralded in community care policy documents (NHS Management Executive 1993).

Thus the changes and shifts in job roles are one major influence on staff development and training strategy. A need exists both to develop new skills and to transfer established skills successfully to new contexts (SSI 1990a), while supporting staff through the destabilizing change processes. Underlying this is a more remedial function (Douglas and Payne 1988) of prioritizing the training needs of long-serving, untrained and unqualified staff in all sectors – statutory, voluntary and independent.

Further influential factors include the emphasis on values and principles underpinning the work, which creates its own set of dilemmas and tensions. Intervening, for example, to support safety and minimize risk entails conflict with principles of maximizing autonomy and self-determination. The challenges to practitioners are complex. Decisions in such circumstances must be informed by balanced reflection, rehearsal for which can be offered through addressing value dilemmas in training. There exists almost a moral imperative for training to help staff to negotiate the value dimension of their work.

'People who are given power and responsibility over others' lives should be prepared, equipped and supervised to discharge those responsibilities adequately [and] must be given the means of learning about what they are doing, how and why' (Douglas and Payne 1988). This applies particularly in the context of the radical value base of empowerment (Smale *et al.* 1993) and the challenging but necessary process of 'turning ourselves inside out' to become centred on users and carers (DoH 1993b).

A third influential factor for the prioritization of training and staff development is that it makes a critical contribution to the quality of services and their positive outcomes for service users. Staff performance is a critical factor in the success of community placements (Mansell and Beasley 1993) but performance quality depends on bottom-up ownership rather than top-down mandates; it must be grown, not imposed. As a means of nurturing that growth staff development is crucial to quality assurance (DoH 1992b).

A final factor influencing training strategy is the importance of its integration with the organizational change required to implement new policy and practice. Training individuals in isolation is unlikely to result in changed practice. 'Clear plans for changes in services and conscious planning and management support for implementing training are also required' (Joseph Rowntree Foundation 1992). The demands of community care policies bring a 'need for changes in attitude and culture throughout agencies' (DoH 1990a). Guidance on training recognizes that training and staff development should be linked explicitly to policy and service development (SSI 1990a), and emphasizes that any implementation agenda must integrate training.

This implies a change in the role of training and staff development sections, towards becoming facilitators of organizational development, working not for the first-order change of grafting new requirements on to old structures but for the second-order change of creating new structures. This envisages radical changes in organizations, their perceptions and how they operate (DoH 1993b).

The influence of these different factors means that training appears to carry a wide-ranging and varied set of responsibilities in relation to successful implementation of community care. Demonstration projects have identified a range of different roles that in practice training is being used to fill:

- dissemination of information to staff about service changes;
- transmission of new philosophies and ways of working required by principles such as user involvement;
- skills acquisition;
- preparation for the emotional and physical demands on staff of community care (Knapp *et al.* 1992).

There is a strong emphasis on values learning and how it should be prioritized in the aims set out for training programmes. CCETSW (1992a), for instance, lists the aims of training in relation to learning disability services as to:

- develop an understanding of individual needs;
- ensure that all staff maintain a holistic view of users;

- reduce the 'clienthood' of users and involve them fully in decision-making about their lives;
- recognize the range of skills staff use to develop relationships, choices, respect, presence and growth for users;
- foster the requisite knowledge, skills and attitudes of staff working collaboratively with users and people from other agencies and disciplines.

There are assumed to be benefits from training to all involved, from staff whose increased skills and knowledge increase motivation and job satisfaction, to agencies who thereby make more efficient use of resources, and service users who receive as high a standard of care as possible (Centre for Policy on Ageing 1990).

The Department of Health (SSI 1991b) emphasizes the importance of training to joint approaches and collaboration across agencies, stressing the importance of identifying common values, skills and knowledge across professional groups and work settings. Training together is promoted as a means of developing a shared philosophy and enhancing collaborative working practices.

Thus training is seen not only as a way to acquire new knowledge and skills, but also as contributing to developing radically different management practices and changing the value perspectives of all involved (Riches and Whitfield 1992), thus carrying responsibility for the large-scale cultural change required for successful policy implementation (Riches 1993). This is a tall order indeed.

Progress on the task is monitored by a community care training strategy group convened by the SSI, with representatives from health, social services, private and voluntary organizations and training bodies, for the purpose of analysing staff training needs, developing training materials and supporting regional joint training initiatives (SSI 1993a). This is mirrored at a local level by the development of joint training groups which are intended to undertake the detailed strategic planning required to differentiate between and plan for the varied approaches needed to tackle inter-agency, multi-agency and single agency issues (DoH 1993b). There is also recognition that training priorities will be linked to the developmental stages of policy implementation during the 1990s – from introducing the changes in the early phases, to managing and consolidating practice and responding to incremental growth at later stages (DoH 1993b).

An early inspection of training strategies in social services departments (SSI 1992d) found room for greater clarity in the strategic planning of training, a need for better coordination between training activity and operational objectives. Recognizing that agencies were attempting to respond to new developments in vocational training and qualification structures, it identified a need for clearer understanding in agencies of the managerial, operational and developmental implications of these, in order to develop the agency infrastructure necessary to support them.

Trends in training

A number of trends have become integral to how training for social care is managed. The underlying theme is that of flexibility – a number of routes to qualification, some based more traditionally in centres of education, others based in employing agencies, or combinations of the two enabling workers to work and prepare for qualifications at the same time. Programmes of learning are increasingly modularized or incorporate distance learning techniques, and owe much to the principle of open learning, with emphasis on control of the programme by the learner (Adams 1993). Credit Accumulation and Transfer, and Accreditation of Prior Learning make it possible for personalized programmes to be undertaken flexibly, at the learner's own pace, and with flexible transfer between programmes to maximize their responsiveness to individual needs and interests.

In-service training is often linked to these structures, carrying credits that can be accumulated and bringing the advantages of more immediate relevance to job roles and responsibilities. Perhaps the most influential trend has been that of emphasizing a worker's observable *performance in the job* as evidence of competency in that job, rather than relying on an assumption of competency derived from academic or professional qualification. If observable performance is what counts, a logical next step is to use this as a basis for awarding qualification. A qualification structure parallel to the more traditional course-based qualification structure has developed, in which people can be assessed as competent in the performance of their job, and receive a qualification, independent of any course of study or training they may have followed. This model has been applied particularly in the vocational job field, and has given rise to the system of National Vocational Qualifications.

The professional qualification arena has, however, also been heavily influenced by the emphasis on observable performance. While qualification at the professional level remains dominated by required programmes of study, such as the Diploma in Social Work, within those programmes the assessment of competence is increasingly dependent upon observed evidence of performance in professional practice, as well as the demonstration of 'knowledge' through academic work. This in turn has brought about a systematization of thinking on what are the components of competent professional task fulfilment, similar to that which has taken place in the vocational field.

The competency model

There are two key concepts within a competency model of professional and vocational job roles. The first is that *workers* can be described as *competent* in the performance of their job. Here competence is the ability to perform in work roles to the standards required (Butler 1991). Competence in a job role depends on workers acquiring and demonstrating key knowledge, skills and values such as those identified by CCETSW (1991b). Within this framework, increasing attention is paid to the clear specification of objectives, the achievement of which can be tangibly demonstrated, rather than abstract aims (Murrell 1993).

The second key concept is that, while a whole set of skills may be needed to perform a particular job, these can be broken down into identifiable elements, recognizable to an observer and thus able to be assessed as they are achieved (Lawler 1994). These *components of competence*, themselves sometimes termed *competencies*, are in effect a functional analysis of professional or vocational job roles, with an emphasis on what people *do* rather than what they *know* because it is the behavioural element in practice rather than the provision of knowledge *per se* that influences whether a person is seen as a good worker (Lawler 1994).

While the competency model has been influential upon thinking about professional training and qualification, it is even more evident in the vocational arena, where the development of a National Vocational Qualifications structure has been dominated by emphasis on assessment of the functional components of vocational job roles.

National vocational qualifications

The National Council for Vocational Qualifications has designed a national framework of qualifications based on standards of occupational competence. These standards are devised from the main functional components of a job *role* rather than of one job or task. This principle has been applied across a wide range of occupational roles, including social care.

The National Occupational Standards for Care (Care Sector Consortium 1992) cover the job roles of those who:

- deliver hands-on care under the supervision, guidance or direction of qualified professional staff;
- deliver hands-on care under the supervision of line managers;
- work in health and social care;
- work in residential, hospital, day and domiciliary care settings.

The Consortium describes the occupational standards as 'quality specifications', defining the quality of performance required in the workplace. They identify a number of key roles in the provision of care, themes which describe the broad desired purposes and outcomes of a worker's involvement in care provision. The key roles in care are:

- support and promote clients' independence in situations of dependency;
- support clients in developing self-sufficiency;
- support clients during specific treatment, therapeutic and development programmes;
- support the maintenance and development of client identity and relationships;
- contribute to the planning, delivery and evaluation of services which provide support and care;
- contribute to the maintenance of an environment for effective care.

Each key role is divided into units describing functions which are associated with the key role and help to achieve it. Each unit is further broken down into elements describing what care workers should be able to do, and performance criteria detailing the behavioural evidence of their competency. Underpinning knowledge is also identified. The whole structure is set within a framework of good practice principles, which make explicit the ethical and moral position taken in the work and must be reflected in every action undertaken. These principles (Care Sector Consortium 1992) place centrally concepts of individuals' rights, equality and anti-discriminatory practice, confidentiality, participation, management of risk, independence, choice and good communication.

The occupational standards contribute to promoting values in social care by identifying a key role of *promoting equality*. This carries the status of being both a separate unit of competence, termed the Value Base Unit, and also a requirement to be evidenced within all functional units. The Value Base Unit is in effect a detailed and explicit statement of what is expected of workers in relation to the principles of good practice. It has its own elements:

- promote anti-discriminatory practice;
- maintain the confidentiality of information;
- promote and support individual rights and choice within service delivery;
- acknowledge individuals' personal beliefs and identity;
- support individuals through effective communication.

Similarly, detailed performance criteria are attached to each element, along with the underpinning knowledge which informs practice.

A National Vocational Qualification in Care may be gained by workers who demonstrate competence in a specified selection of units from the Standards, and may be achieved at level two or level three. All qualifications must comprise a core requirement, which includes the Value Base Unit plus a set of specified Functional Units, together with an Endorsement made up of a number of functional units relevant to the particular work setting of the worker.

The introduction of NVQs, with their emphasis on demonstrated competence on the job, has been accompanied by a radical reframing of the relationship between training as input and competence as output (Kelly *et al.* 1990). While standards of competence are highly detailed and heavily prescribed, the routes that workers take to prepare for demonstrating competence are very flexible and do not assume a causal link between training and qualification. The award of a qualification is independent of training (CCETSW 1992b) and candidates could, in theory, apply to have their competence assessed without having undergone any formal training. In practice, many in-service training and college-based courses are targeted on specific units and aim to prepare workers for assessment. The assessment structure is prescribed by the NCVQ, which authorizes awarding bodies (in the case of social care, CCETSW and City and Guilds) to regulate the arrangements and make the awards. Any agency wishing to assess its workers for care awards must be able to offer an adequate range of opportunity for demonstrating competence and adequate mechanisms for the assessment and support of candidates. Common interpretation of the standards will be monitored by internal verifiers. The awarding body will also appoint an external verifier to monitor issues of standardization across centres, resource levels, learning opportunities and appeals.

Within the National Standards is guidance on how evidence of competence may be gathered and presented. Direct observation of workers' activities by their assessor is emphasized, but supplementary methods, such as role play, case study, oral and written reports and testimony from others, may also be used. In essence the assessment procedures are designed to test three aspects of a worker's functioning:

- skills in the performance of tasks;
- ability to apply principles and values;
- understanding of why those tasks are performed, in terms of both underpinning knowledge and organizational policy and procedures (Harvey and Tisdall 1992).

The design and implementation of NVQs in Care incorporate many of the themes identified earlier in the training and staff development arena, the keynotes being flexibility and job role relevance. Workers may choose the awards most suitable to their own work setting, progress at their own speed and include learning acquired in prior contexts. Credit Accumulation and Transfer is also integral to the system. Workers may collect as many awards at any level as they wish.

Considerable work is being undertaken to link the National Standards at their differing levels to the requirements of qualification that employers might impose for recruitment or progression in paid employment, or might offer to staff as in-service qualification opportunities. Additionally, further developments will clarify the relationship between NVQs and existing awards, such as BTEC, and between 'vocational' and 'professional' levels of competency in social care, such as that recognized by the Diploma in Social Work.

While there are problems of implementation which centre on resource levels in agencies and the relevance and availability of preparatory training, there are potentially several benefits in the longer term, identified as (Harvey and Tisdall 1992):

- introducing an effective quality control mechanism in the workplace;
- enhancing the importance of supervision;
- offering a systematic staff development structure for organizations to follow;
- overturning the notion that care work equates with common sense and commitment, and thus contributing to a revaluing of care provision tasks.

Additionally, the emphasis on flexibility offers the potential for experience and competence gained in unpaid work to be recognized, thus extending opportunities of access to qualification to women who have not held status in the paid labour market but whose contribution to social care provision has been marked (Butler 1991).

The problems with competency

While the competency model has been widely influential upon training and staff development, it has not been universally welcomed as unproblematic. Broadly, criticisms come from two positions:

- that the notion of competency as translated into performance indicators inadequately describes what occurs in an encounter, either between service users and workers, or between workers and those assessing their competence;

- that the notion of worker competency does not adequately reflect other factors that impinge on the encounter, external to the worker and service user but none the less influential.

There is criticism that the focus on skills and observable behaviour gives insufficient weight to the importance of values in social care, and inadequately reflects the recognized impact of staff attitudes on the quality of life of care consumers (Centre for Policy on Ageing 1990). The importance of such recognition is reinforced by findings of sometimes very negative attitudes among care staff, amounting to overt judgementalism and discriminatory behaviour (DoH 1993c). The personal triggers that may exist for staff in social care work must be acknowledged when the situations encountered interact with workers' own personal histories and characteristics, leading to responses such as denial, rejection or idealization (Segal 1991). Even basic definitions, and how workers understand and interpret them, are driven by value assumptions and models which the notion of worker competency as observed in practice does not make explicit. The NVQ response to such criticism has been to develop the Value Base Unit, with its emphasis on anti-discriminatory practice, confidentiality, rights and choice. Performance criteria for the functional units, however, despite the requirement that the value base be demonstrated throughout, do not reflect the permeation of values that is required to establish their centrality. A further criticism is of the mechanistic and reductionist, technical way in which complex processes are described. This 'recipe book' thinking (Wilson 1992) fails to engage with tensions, dilemmas and complexities in the job or with questioning and understanding of the nature of tasks being undertaken. Competencies, because they are derived from functional analyses of a job rather than from studies of what effective practitioners actually do, can represent only generalizations of what is done in practice, and are too mechanistic to represent the unique combinations of factors at work in individual situations (Lawler 1994). Nor can they represent the different contributions arising from the diversity of experience represented in a mixed and varied workforce of the differing interpretations that diverse gender, race and class perspectives might bring to key criteria against which performance is judged. These criteria, based on common-sense assumptions of what is good and desirable, will inevitably reflect the norms and perspectives of dominant groups in society (Kemshall 1993).

The components of a worker's approach to given tasks are also far more complex than an emphasis on observable behaviour and skills would suggest. Knowledge and values enter in subtle ways, not as separate factors but as integral processes: knowledge in action becomes 'know-how' (Schön 1993), knowing that is inherent in the action rather than a separate 'testable' factor. The relationship between knowledge and practice is not a linear one in which the former is applied to the latter, but is more circular and integrated, the one informing the other in a process of evolution (Secker 1993).

Also missing from the competency model, yet vital to social care practice where practitioners will encounter 'greater diversity than that for which [they] can be prepared' (England 1986), is any focus on the ability to transfer learning from prior experience to new and unpredictable situations (Walmsley *et al.* 1993). The ability to engage in the reflection that enables transfer of learning is essential in particular for the development of anti-discriminatory practice which cannot be achieved through reliance on technical skills alone (Humphries 1993). The danger in this omission is that it encourages prescription of thinking, feeling and behaving in situations which actually require flexibility, use of self and discretion (Kelly *et al.* 1990). Training based on such a model risks divorcing people from their humanity, teaching them to listen rather than to hear; to record, not to understand; to diagnose and treat, not to feel (Stewart 1991).

What attracts concern is the model's inability to deal with intangible factors which cannot be observed in behaviour and are indeed difficult to describe in words. Functional analysis of job roles, in attempting to divide a key role into its component parts, fails to allow that the experience of an encounter between two people is more than the sum of its constituent parts; that two workers can perform the same functions yet only one of them be experienced as empowering.

Concern with the content of *what* is done can lead to neglect of process (Coulshed 1993), which essentially is what defines the quality of a relationship and establishes its importance as a contribution to professional effectiveness. In the context of concerns about the recognition within the competency model of important but intangible processes, problems also arise with using observed behaviour as the key to identifying how far workers achieve standards of competency in their practice. There are two issues here. One is the wide margin of error inherent in using observed behaviour to assess competence, which has to include dimensions of knowledge and values alongside skills. Not only is behaviour constrained by many factors additional to a worker's ability, but the same behaviour can have various different meanings (Kelly *et al.* 1990). The second is that what is observed is filtered through the subjective bias of the observer, whose own personal processes and values, in addition to the context in which the work is undertaken, impinge upon what is seen and how it is judged. The logical extension of this analysis is that competence becomes merely the 'point at which the supervisee's performance fits with the subjective view of the assessor and the organisational goals of the agency' (Kemshall 1993), a notion that is particularly problematic in relation to the assessment of values and attitudes.

The second category of objections to the competency model reflects concerns that its focus is too individual; that competency is presented as a personal Everest to be climbed if one is fit, strong and persistent; and that individual worker competence is the key factor in the achievement of key role objectives with service users. What this individual focus fails to allow for is the 'inheritance factor' (Lawler 1994), the impact of other people or situations on the user's situation, the organizational culture in which the worker operates, the political context in which the organization performs its work. Worker competence depends not just upon a personal framework of knowledge, skills and values, but also upon the level of support for it in the organizational context which provides the environmental factors that nurture and foster good practice to reach the standards set (Moonie and Newlyn

1990). This recognition, that competence is not merely an individual phenomenon, has resulted in attention being given to the notion of the competent workplace (Pottage and Evans 1992), where the culture and policies support competent job performance rather than militate against it. The notion of a competent workplace requires further exploration, not just because of its potential impact upon competent practice in workers, but also because an organization's ethos and culture is central to how core values are integrated within social care practice.

The competent organization

Workers will experience difficulty empowering and valuing others when they do not feel powerful and valued (Read and Wallcraft 1992). Workers required or wanting to work in an open and empowering way will experience difficulties when their organization does not support them or, worse, is experienced by them as closed and oppressive. There are several ways in which staff feel constrained by their employing organization. At a resource level practitioners frequently feel asked to undertake a role with insufficient time or resources to fulfil it either to their own satisfaction or to the standards required in policy and practice guidance. The demoralization of staff attempting to undertake needs-led assessments in the knowledge that resources are unavailable to meet the needs illustrates this point. This is often a frustration shared by managers and workers alike, although there are clearly situations in which workers feel oppressed by their managers, as a result of ethos and style rather than resource levels. Contributing to this are situations where workers are subject to high demands but enjoy low autonomy in their ability to manoeuvre between those demands owing to what is experienced as excessive control and regulation by authoritarian management practices and attitudes; where management relations with staff are characterized by suspicion and blame, enemies in adversarial encounter rather than allies of staff in a common endeavour.

At a more subtle level the organization and structuring of the agency's work can deny staff what they want and need for work satisfaction. For instance, an analysis of strict nursing routines in hospital wards (Menzies 1970), designed to defend against powerful anxieties generated by the work, protected nurses from emotional closeness with patients but left them with unresolved stress. The perceived masculinization of management (Grimwood and Popplestone 1993) is influential here, with problems arising from the identification of management with instrumental 'masculine' qualities which divorces it from expressive roles associated with caring and the integration of emotion or feeling. The status differentiation perceivable within vocational and professional roles also carries a gender dimension, in that the feminine roles of *caring for* people are carried out under the direction of masculine planning and care management roles. This distortion of management brings about a self-fulfilling effect in that women will opt out or be excluded from management positions, or their management style may go unappreciated (Grimwood and Popplestone 1993).

A further example of how workers are not empowered lies in how organizations recognize their status. Social care providers will often be among the lower-paid staff with the least favourable conditions and status in their organization. Individual competency has to be supported by demonstrable recognition of the value of the work being undertaken (Mitchell 1993).

What, then, might a competent organization be like to work in? First, the organizational change required must be recognized for the agency's structure and ethos to be one which supports workers in competent practice led by the values of empowerment. User involvement and partnership in planning requires participative management, delegated responsibility and devolved decision-making (Smale *et al.* 1993). This requires a culture in which power is an overt agenda, and where recognition of and feedback on how it is used, both within the organization and between it and those who use its services, is permitted and encouraged. This will entail the development of management styles which foster and promote a more egalitarian culture, which are democratic rather than autocratic (Handy 1985) and which reflect and value more feminine styles of management, identified (Loden 1985) as including the use of power to empower, challenging hierarchical roles and boundaries, non-adversarial approaches to conflict, intuitive as well as rational problem-solving, an emphasis on teamwork and the prominence of interpersonal skills such as listening and empathy. The organization's own employment practices are crucial here, with positive attention given to the position of black workers, women, disabled people and others commonly discriminated against in employment.

Second, competent organizations ensure clarity of goal setting and engage staff at all levels with these goals. Broad goals must also be translated into detailed objectives: impact objectives, relating to the agency's purposes and the specific effects it is intended to have; service objectives, concerning the ways in which the impact can be achieved; and logistical objectives, concerning the structures needed to support the services (Bovaird and Mallinson 1988). Clear policy statements, up-to-date procedures and staff guidance on practice are key features (SSI 1992a), as are clarity and agreement about standards (DoH 1992b) and the outcome measures that will be used as part of the quality assurance framework. Within this broad framework of goal setting, a competent organization will emphasize and prioritize objectives which reflect a commitment to integrating values within its structures and practices. Anti-discriminatory practice, for example, requires change not just at the level of individual attitude and behaviour, but an organizational infrastructure to provide policy, support, consultation and representation procedures (Ahmad-Aziz *et al.* 1992).

Additionally, the way in which an organization develops its objectives is crucial to the empowerment of staff within the system. An organizational development approach to change entails staff working together to identify the objectives, strategies, values and role definitions to be promoted by the organization in pursuit of its broad aims (LBTC 1992) and is important in developing the sense of ownership throughout the organization necessary for successful implementation.

Third, organizational competency lies in the arrangements made to support staff in performing its objectives. If care is organized to maximize positive contact between staff and service users, a potentially high level of stress and anxiety will result for workers within such contact. This arises not only from the intensity of personal interaction that will be experienced, but also from the awareness of competing priorities in primary tasks and of conflicting values that may be applied. A number of mechanisms make an important contribution here. Supervision ensures accountability and enhances performance through constructive feedback and by ensuring access to more intensive staff care if required. A safe environment will enable staff to express doubt, undertake necessary learning, experiment and innovate. These are processes to which group support, affiliation and problem-solving can positively contribute (Hanmer and Statham 1988; Makin *et al.* 1989). They require organizations to support and encourage such affiliation.

Staff must also feel empowered to voice concerns they may hold. Evidence indicates high levels of concern among practitioners about the extent to which organizations adhere to the values that should underpin their work, such that an organization, 'Public Concern at Work', exists to support and protect from victimization people struggling to expose malpractice (Erlichman 1994). Staff face considerable difficulties, as speaking out often involves questioning the organizational culture, established ways of working or colleagues' practice (Kelly 1993). High costs have been paid by people speaking out in organizations which respond defensively. A competent organization encourages feedback from staff and will offer guidelines and procedures to enable people to express concern without breaking confidentiality and risking their own employment (Sone 1992).

The 'competency' of an organization is, therefore, a vital part of the framework that supports the delivery of effective services. Without such competency, an individual worker's knowledge, skills and values, important though they are, will not achieve their maximum potential. A danger also exists that training individuals will be seen as the preferred means of achieving required changes, when in fact policy and organizational changes are necessary. Training and staff development programmes must be fully integrated, therefore, with the organizational development agenda to ensure consistency of priorities and to maximize the contribution of each.

Challenges to training and staff development

Successfully integrating training and staff development with organizational change is just one of the challenges that exist in training for social care. Another is the balance between the separate functions of *training* and *staff development*, which, though linked, may usefully be distinguished from each other. Staff development covers those 'processes used to assist people's abilities to learn, change attitudes and behaviour, and to improve performance within a given job or occupation' (Douglas and Payne 1988). Thus most of what workers do may be deemed staff development, provided it is linked into a systematic framework for evaluating performance and identifying areas for development. Work experiences that are subsequently examined and reflected upon, perhaps in supervision, observation visits, discussions with colleagues and other agencies, reading, study and course work, are all activities that contribute to staff development. Training may contribute, as a structured learning experience set aside from everyday work activity, and aiming to enhance knowledge, skills and values necessary for work competency, or perhaps as a required component of a route to qualification. Training is most effective when offered as part of an overall staff development strategy, which itself will derive from organizational change goals.

A further challenge lies in determining the balance between generic and specialist learning. Insofar as community care policy has a broad application to differing groups of people, united by their need or wish for services rather than other unifying factors, certain aspects of learning are truly generic: the policy context, the value base, the mechanisms for accessing and providing services. Alongside this must be placed the particular learning needs of staff working with people who have a more narrowly defined range of needs, or whose role focuses on a specific area of users' lives. The danger here, while the specialist need doubtless exists, lies in then restricting professional attention to that one need or aspect of life, a tendency to categorize people to fit professional perceptions rather than take a holistic view (SSI 1993b). In the context of changing professional roles and uncertainty about the future of key aspects of social care provision, there must be further clarification of the impact of policy implementation on job roles before the direction of specialist training becomes clear.

Another challenge lies in negotiating the balance between assisting people to develop practical, functional skills, and promoting knowledge and values learning. The danger of attempting an overt focus on values learning, as Marsh and Fisher (1992) demonstrate in relation to partnership, is that workers commonly avoid engaging with a learning process by relying on a 'we do that already' response. A major contribution that training and staff development can make here is to render values tangible, to consider the behavioural evidence that workers are performing their tasks from a required value base, to ask for answers to the question 'how will service users *know* you believe it is important to practise anti-oppressively; what will they see you doing, hear you saying?' This is particularly important when learning about anti-oppressive practice, which entails unlearning deeply ingrained ideas and behaviour learned in early childhood and thus is likely to encounter some resistance. Being able to focus learning on the behaviours and tasks required in the workplace, and focusing on practical understandings besides conceptual understanding, can greatly assist this process and render it more successful as a learning experience (Ahmad 1991).

Next, the development of the market economy in social care provision is bringing in providers from an independent sector about which relatively little is known concerning the amount or quality of training available to staff. What is known (Staton 1993) indicates a focus in training on practical tasks, and an assumption that sensitive individualized care would 'come naturally' if staff with the right attitudes were appointed. Training is seen as an optional extra, not as an investment. Market forces may need to be influential here, as local authorities take initiatives in specifying required levels of training and qualification in their purchasing contracts.

The final challenge is ensuring that how learning opportunities are experienced is consistent with the value base that underpins their content. This is pertinent in three ways. First, in constructing learning experiences which prioritize values such as partnership and empowerment, the involvement and contribution of service users must be maximized, in both planning and participating in training and other staff development opportunities. Such involvement must reflect careful thought and negotiation about its purposes and boundaries, to avoid dangers of involving people in ways that are tokenistic or exploitative. Such involvement brings a number of strong contributions enabling workers to access information not available from any other source, allowing, for example, space and opportunity for experimentation with partnership models and with new relationships which challenge assumptions behind why social care provision is made (Biggs 1993).

Second, a further translation of the partnership principle into training is the degree to which the goals, content and processes of training are negotiated *with* participants as opposed to being imposed, and are able to draw out and build on their experiences and strengths (Braye and Preston-Shoot 1993a). Third, learning experiences offered should provide opportunities for people to learn in an environment where they will not be subject to oppressive behaviour from others. This involves clear understandings about the permissions that exist in any context to share views and express opinions, along with a commitment to ensuring that those views and opinions are shared constructively in the process of learning and not used to oppress others in that same learning situation.

Key factors

Major changes have taken place and developments will continue in social care training as agencies, educational bodies, trainers and individual staff members progressively engage with new systems, and the systems themselves are refined to reflect feedback from implementation. None the less, five key features can be isolated that distinguish good quality staff development provision. The first is an emphasis on the integration of staff and organizational development. If training is to contribute to the change process it must be integral from the beginning, integrating individual, team, organizational and inter-organizational development with the pursuit of new occupational tasks (LBTC 1992). To be effective agents of change, trainers must build alliances with managers, operational staff, users, other agencies and accrediting bodies (LBTC 1992), an interactive approach that will coordinate and structure the management of organizational change.

The second is that training and staff development strategy must be built on systematic analysis of needs and priorities, itself informed by considerations which move beyond a sole focus on the individual skills of workers. One model (K. Williams 1991) proposes three influences, with priorities lying in the area of overlap between them: service users' needs and what is required to meet these; the 'personal profiling' strengths and weaknesses of staff; and the priorities of the organization. Others (for example, CCETSW 1992a; NISW/NEC 1993) propose models for systematization of the process, from needs analysis through to planning for linking this to aims, objectives and outcomes. The analysis must cover all organizational levels and be able to address the needs not just of specific groups of workers but also of workers and managers together, identifying and developing their mutual contributions to quality service development. The process must also be participative, creating dialogue between the various interests represented in the organization and ensuring links between various service sectors.

The third key feature is an approach to learning that borrows some aspects of adult learning principles, for instance (Douglas and Payne 1988) that the themes of learning are based in situations familiar to people, are rooted in experience or the potential range of experience available to staff, and have immediate relevance to practice in the workplace. Such an approach is based on the belief that 'significant learning occurs through the creation of knowledge from and the transformation of knowledge into actual work experience' (Pottage and Evans 1992). This is entirely consistent with a staff development approach which identifies learning opportunities across a much wider spectrum than simply direct training, and which requires direct training, where given, to address the work context explicitly. A further influence from adult learning is the self-directed nature of new qualification structures, emphasizing the flexibility for individual programmes of modularization, credit accumulation and transfer, and accreditation of prior learning.

There is, however, a dimension to add to the adult learning focus, one which is particularly important in the context of values learning. The non-negotiable components of learning must be identified, in work roles where demonstration of competency must include evidence of anti-discriminatory practice. Attention must be given to the processes which can affect learning: the need for support and encouragement to confront personal values and to change behaviour that is deeply ingrained; the recognition of past and current discriminatory and devaluing experiences and of power dynamics in workplace relationships, which can act as barriers and must be addressed (Inner London Probation Service undated).

The fourth key feature is monitoring and evaluating the impact of training and staff development programmes. Evaluation has traditionally been focused upon the quality of *input* – of the course, the programme, the learning opportunity. Any focus on outcome has been in respect of an individual's skill development or assessed competency. There is increasing recognition, consistent with the emphasis on aims and objectives linked with organizational change priorities, of the need to evaluate the outcome of training and staff development experiences in terms of their impact on service provision (SSI 1993e), and of the importance of including such evaluation at the outset of planning so that it becomes an integral part of the process.

Finally, agencies must develop notions of quality and standards in training and staff development. There are several ways to tackle this, most commonly through lists of key principles to be observed (for instance, LBTC 1992), which draw attention to issues of:

• user and community involvement in training development;
• creative design of training, using a range of techniques;

- cross-sector, multidiscplinary training;
- anti-discriminatory and ethnically sensitive training;
- commitment to quality assurance;
- training for all levels of staff, including cross-level;
- integrating training into accreditation systems;
- senior management endorsement of training as a vehicle for change;
- planning and reviewing training, assessing individual needs regularly.

The problem with principles is that they must be made more specific before they can be termed standards. The SSI (1992d) has begun this task, and proposes more specific requirements, such as the presence of written policy and the identification of resources. An alternative to the generation of lists is a single model (Boyes 1993) which takes five key desirable concepts – appropriateness, effectiveness, acceptability, equity and efficiency – and requires them to be demonstrated in the three key stages of planning, delivery and outcomes of staff development. Such a model enables flexibility in setting standards while ensuring that key aspects are covered.

Exercise 3.1.   Think about how you learned to do the job you are doing now. How much of that learning took place in your workplace? What learning opportunities were there? How could you make these learning opportunities useful to you now?

Exercise 3.2.   Consider a situation in which you were learning something important. What was helpful and what unhelpful to your learning? How could your learning have been made easier?

Exercise 3.3.   Describe a critical incident that took place at work recently, something that was challenging or difficult. Identify the knowledge, skills and values that helped you deal with it. Apply these qualities to a current problem that you are feeling uncertain about how to tackle, thereby transferring your learning. What knowledge, skills and values would help you deal with such situations in a different way?

Exercise 3.4.   Choose six things that your employing organization can do to empower you to be competent. Which of these are already in place? What action could you initiate concerning those not yet in place?

Exercise 3.5.   Identify the skills that you require for your job. Which of these do you feel confident about? Which do you feel would benefit from further training and staff development activity? What sources of help exist, what opportunities for development can you access? When will you do this?

Exercise 3.6.   Take a training or staff development activity in which you have been involved. Using the chart below (Boyes 1993), identify the criteria by which you would assess the quality of that experience: how it was planned, your experience of it and the outcomes it has had for you.

	Planning	Delivery	Outcome
Appropriateness			
Effectiveness			
Acceptability			
Equity			
Efficiency			

Part II Conflicting imperatives

and practice dilemmas:

finding creative

and coherent solutions

The opening chapters analysed the policy and legal mandates, the professional value base, and the training and organizational environment within which social care practice operates. This context is not unproblematic. Community care reforms point towards a different relationship between social care agencies and users. Goals and services should be user-led rather than profession-dominated, founded on a partnership approach and reflecting user needs and wishes rather than provider preferences. The user's voice is to be stronger, but how strong? Talk of empowerment and partnership, of needs-led provision and choice, may sound impressive but conceals very real dilemmas within social care relationships and obscures the different meanings and scope which various stakeholders will apply. In this the key questions 'why' and 'how' are in danger of becoming lost.

There are crucial questions. When should practitioners intervene and with what level of service: the minimum intervention necessary or an optimum provision? By what process should the focus of involvement be determined and how should the interests or conflicting expectations of different stakeholders be balanced? What should practice emphasize when there exist professional concerns about power and inequality: about the mismatch between levels of need and resources, and between user and professional definitions of needs; and about the disempowering nature of much professional involvement? How can practitioners negotiate the twin requirements to empower users and to gatekeep resources?

Legislation and policy, in emphasizing the language of partnership and empowerment, may have resonated with professional preoccupations, but achieving a different relationship may prove elusive. Different variations of care management have appeared, prioritizing budgetary planning, advocacy to enable users to negotiate through the social care system and empowerment to change the system in line with user definitions of need (Biggs and Weinstein 1991). The legal mandate and services prompted by it continue to represent dominant beliefs, to elevate individual adaptation and change above the social dimensions of problems which individuals encounter, and to be experienced as oppressive and controlling (Grimwood and Popplestone 1993). Where 'the problem' lies is an assumption yet to be challenged effectively.

Achieving a different, empowering relationship between users and social care workers requires a critical understanding of the assumptions and ideologies which underpin social care, and of the complexities, tensions and dilemmas which result. These will be grouped thematically and explored by reference to the knowledge-base which assists understanding and points to the implications for empowering practice, the skills required to negotiate the choices inherent in specific situations. The end point is practice which translates understanding into action at individual, organizational and political levels within social care. This requires an analysis which clarifies the relationship between law, policy and practice, and provides a critical edge concerning how the law and policy help or hinder professional endeavours, and promote or constrain equality for people vulnerable through age, disability or illness. That analysis, with practice as its end point, is the focus in this section.

4 Conflicts of interest

in social care

Two major challenges face social care professionals. One revolves around determining who or what controls the provision and quality of services: people's needs, their rights or resource availability. What is prioritized will influence subsequent practice decisions, while the potential clash between the three elements will be exacerbated further by conflicts of interest: between users and those whose caring role brings rights and needs of their own; between users and professionals; between different professional groups and agencies. The second challenge lies in determining who makes which decisions about people's lives, the individual or the state, and by reference to what values. The focus here is on the competency in decision-making of people who use services and the nature of compulsory powers available for their care and treatment. Who should decide what happens to a vulnerable person? Does the person have decision-making autonomy or should others assume responsibility and, if so, for what purpose and using what criteria?

Such is the complexity of these questions and the different perspectives through which they may be answered that consensus is elusive about what should be done, when and how. Proposals, for instance, to electronically tag confused older people in residential care are variously welcomed as evidence of a caring approach or condemned as interference with and a violation of fundamental civil liberties. Similar controversy greeted proposals to provide new legal powers to social workers to protect dependent and vulnerable adults (Law Commission 1993). As in child protection, different incidents prompt calls for tighter legal controls or for the reassertion of individual rights against negligent or heavy-handed authorities.

Neither the NHS and Community Care Act 1990 nor subsequent policy guidance recognizes or addresses these tensions: the competing demands of welfare, protection and rights; the competing ideologies of *laissez-faire* and patriarchy, state paternalism and user rights; the dilemmas of developing flexible and responsive services while gatekeeping to regulate demand. Indeed, policy specifically endorses conflicting priorities (Parsloe 1993), including user choice and budgetary controls.

Wide variations in service provision result, with calls for legally enforceable entitlement rights (Brindle 1993). Another outcome is the division of people with equal needs into deserving and undeserving categories, both in practice and in policy, a phenomenon which contributes to the corruption of care (Wardhaugh and Wilding 1993) when some groups become seen as somehow not fully human.

The juxtaposition of different interests or priorities for action, as if without conflict between them, results in rights to and needs for services becoming entangled with questions of resource availability. Professional values and assessments, together with user definitions of need, are vulnerable to collusion between local and central government. To protect some limited autonomy for local government, and the welfare professions therein, radical approaches to empowering rights-based services are replaced by practices which limit user participation in decision-making, promote an individualized focus on need and omit reference to how social structures create disadvantage and perpetuate inequalities (Borsay 1986; Brady 1992; Cornwell 1992/3). Professionals cannot be trusted to act in people's best interests (Wilding 1982).

Juxtaposing different interests and priorities for action without clarifying what the terminology means for practice reinforces rather than challenges the power of inherited ideas and practices. Moreover, community care can simultaneously be supported because it empowers users and demystifies professionalism, yet promotes economic solutions to social problems through informal caring networks (Levick 1992). Since the extent to which need assessment should be separate from resource questions remains unclear, and since what needs should or must be met remains uncertain, the relationship between needs and resources is confused rather than debated. Responsibility for confusion about rights, needs and resources, and for the catalogue of complaints (Cervi 1993a) about inadequate information on services, restricted criteria for assessment and service eligibility, and the absence of a legal right to assessment, can be diverted away from policy towards alleged weaknesses in local authorities. Furthermore, key values – privacy, dignity, independence, choice, rights and fulfilment (DoH 1989c) – will only guide practitioners through dilemmas such as balancing risk-taking with protection when the policy mandate is clear and fully resourced.

Not surprisingly, for those whose basic human rights, such as to live and travel where they choose, have been infringed and diminished by social and economic structures, dependence on imposed assessment procedures and segregated worker-inspired facilities (Bynoe et al. 1991), the emphasis on needs-led assessments, choice and partnership rings hollow. Equality remains elusive for many citizens. This chapter proposes a critical questioning and fundamental rethink of the relationship between law, policy and practice. It argues for clarity of meaning and clear entitlements within consolidated legislation that enables people to address the social problems which are expressed through individual need and to achieve equality of opportunity, independence and dignity. This involves codifying rights to services based on people's unique needs and expressed wishes, and promoting the greatest possible self-determination on the basis of informed choice (Mind 1983).

Exercise 4.1.   How would you define a quality service? Who or what should control the quality and provision of service? How would you define need? What rights would you stress? Who is competent to make what decisions? How would your agency approach these questions, and how does this approach compare with how you have defined a quality service?

Theme 1: who or what controls the provision and quality of services?

Central to social care provision is the concept of a quality service but the components of, and the routes to achieving, quality are complex (Braye and Preston-Shoot 1994).

People should have the services that meet their *needs*.

People have a *right* to good quality services.

People should have services which make cost-effective and efficient use of *resources*.

All three statements reflect government rhetoric on social care but there is no guidance on the relationship between needs, rights and resources, on the dilemmas and tensions posed in implementing these potentially conflicting mandates.

Need

Being '*in need* of care and attention' is a passport to provision (NAA 1948). There is duty to '*assess the need* to make arrangements' on behalf of people covered by section 29 of the National Assistance Act 1948, and to give practical assistance '*where satisfied it is necessary*' (CSDPA 1970). A disabled person or his or her carer may request an *assessment of needs* (DPA 1986). Local authorities must 'assess an *individual's need* for services and . . . decide whether the need calls for the provision of services' (NHSCCA 1990). The duty to provide after-care to individuals (MHA 1983) ceases when authorities are satisfied that they are no longer *in need* of such services.

How need is defined is less clear. The Disabled Persons (SCR) Act (section 4) appears to endorse *felt* and *expressed need*, since users and carers may request an assessment, which local authorities must undertake. The NHS and Community Care Act (section 47), by contrast, promotes *prescribed need* whereby professionals determine whether an assessment is required. In both cases, however, professionals assess need, with no guarantee that users' definitions of their needs will form the basis of any care package. Rather, local authorities may use *normative* (set standards) or *comparative need* (who is or is not receiving services) definitions (Bradshaw 1972) when deciding if services are necessary.

Moreover, law and policy incorporate different approaches to establishing and responding to need (see Barclay Report 1982; Fox Harding 1991). A 'safety-net approach' envisages a minimal state role, complementing informal networks provided by individuals, families and communities. State intervention is regarded as inimical to people's welfare but, where necessary, is characterized by authoritarianism, as in compulsory care measures (section 47, NAA 1948). This *laissez-faire* approach reflects a mistrust of state intervention and a belief in the law's limitations, evidenced in the absence of legislation to protect vulnerable, abused adults. It is patriarchal in its assumption of family and community provision, an assumption which is firmly entrenched in the ideology of the NHS and Community Care Act 1990, where care *in* the community has been replaced with care *by* the community, yet without resources to change the gendered divisions in caring and thereby intensifying the inequalities experienced by women (Baldwin and Twigg 1991).

The 'welfare state approach' envisages comprehensive services within which the state retains ultimate control but with users and other service providers having some involvement in decision-making. Its emphasis on individual pathology and faith in the state to provide protection and care (MHA 1983; section 47, NAA 1948; case law on consent to medical treatment) embodies paternalism; its emphasis on supportive intervention through service provision to reduce the impact of older age, disability and ill-health, and to promote people's welfare (section 2, CSDPA 1970; section 45, HSPHA 1968), represents defence of individuals and families.

These legal mandates view need in individual and, primarily, medical terms (Barton 1993). Individuals are expected to adapt to society; the social environment is not expected to adjust to the needs and aspirations of disabled or older people. Needs are seen to reside in personal rather than structural deficiencies, even though the latter restrict life chances and impair social participation. Thus, the very concept of need becomes disabling (Sapey and Hewitt 1991) because disabled and older people are seen as people in need rather than people whose rights to resources are being denied or rationed.

Furthermore, these approaches are professionally led and dominated. The *laissez-faire* approach assumes a one-dimensional power relationship (Rees 1991) between users and practitioners. Practitioners control the agenda, with compliance demanded within assumed agreement on the dominant values by which society is organized. The professional and the political are separated. The welfare state approach assumes a two-dimensional relationship which is reformist but within officially sanctioned procedures. Users may participate in expressing choice but decision-making power about which options are suitable to enable individuals to achieve, maintain or restore an acceptable level of independence or quality of life resides with professionals (DoH 1991b). Social structures are not questioned. The emphasis remains on what people can or cannot do, and therefore have needs in respect of, rather than on what people are prevented from doing by the environment within which they live. Services are provided not because people have an active right but because a passive need has been established. The further one moves from the dominant image of competency and self-provision, the fewer rights one has. To be old, disabled or poor is to be less of a citizen (Braye and Preston-Shoot 1992a).

Such needs-based approaches have been criticized for encouraging passivity and dependence (Illich 1975; Smale 1983), for imposing on individuals the values of an oppressive and discriminatory society, and for being ineffective and unethical (Mayer and Timms 1970; Llewelyn 1987) because they impose a definition of 'best interests' rather than act on how users define their reality. They represent a considerable departure from a user-centred approach based on devolved power and decision-making to users. Their implications for intervention and service provision are increasingly rejected by disabled people (Borsay 1986; Barnes 1992; Mullender 1992/3), who argue for an overhaul of the language and scope of the legislation, and for a rights-based, anti-oppressive approach to needs. This would emphasize autonomy and independence, focus on restrictive and disabling environments, and prioritize social change rather than individual adjustment. Care plans and services would challenge and minimize the effects of structural inequalities and restrictive social attitudes and arrangements.

Need, therefore, is not self-evident. Nor do policy and practice yet have a coherent, clear and detailed theory of need on which to base assessments and standards of provision (Doyal and Gough 1991). The statement that care packages must be needs-led, tailored to assessed need (DoH 1989a; SSI 1993d), omits more than it conveys. This disempowers users and practitioners seeking to assert rights or to use unmet needs to inform community care plans. The emphasis on individual need masks common social needs and obscures the problems which arise for groups of people from the operation of social norms and policies. It renders over-optimistic the claim (Smale et al. 1993) that a needs-led approach will prevent stereotyping in assessments. It jeopardizes the ability of services to improve the quality of life and of the environment (Baldwin 1986).

Service users' needs remain a judgement for professionals. Their wishes are not determinative, either in defining need or in determining how it will be met. They do not control the process. Indeed, professionals must judge how users may participate (DoH 1991b), a paternalism which directly contradicts the principle and experience that people can speak authoritatively about their own needs. This professional domination leaves people feeling isolated and blamed, their needs not understood (SSI 1991c). The assessment may lose sight of life experience (Baldwin 1986; CCETSW 1992a). Ambiguity exists concerning what comprehensive assessments should include. User-perceived needs, race and culture, and housing, for example, should be included (DoH 1991b). However, emotional needs may be considered irrelevant (Parsloe 1993); the distinction between wants and needs remains unclear; assessment may fail to acknowledge cultural pressures which have disabling effects on women, disabled people and minority groups (SSI 1993b); and housing need may be overlooked although suitable housing can reduce or even remove social care needs (Arnold et al. 1993).

Expressed and felt needs may also be recast as wishes and preferences, devalued so that local authorities may avoid their legal responsibility to meet assessed needs. Since authorities also have discretion concerning eligibility criteria for services (when services should be provided) and how assessed needs are best met (type of service to provide), a conflict of interest emerges: care packages must be the best available way to meet needs but must be cost-effective for the local authority and within available resources. This require-ment is undisturbed by questions of risk, compulsory powers, dilemmas when resources influence available services and whether the services avail-able are what people regard as relevant. The purchaser–provider split masks these tensions by implying the possibility of separating questions of need from resources, and by ignoring the practice dilemmas of humanitarianism versus economics, professionalism versus organizational procedures (Braye and Preston-Shoot 1992a).

The muddle is apparent, finally, in guidance which simultaneously re-quires local authorities to decide what is an acceptable quality of life for users (DoH 1989a) while advocating (SSI 1993b) the need to change and redefine the professional role *from* an expert definer of need and gatekeeper of services *to* a resource which people may negotiate to use as *they* choose.

Rights

Exercise 4.2.   List the rights which you believe people have and should have when (a) negotiating social care provision and (b) receiving social care. Note any differences between the two lists.

Exercise 4.3.   On an average day, to what extent do you have access to choice, personal and professional networks, employment, transport, personal relationships and income? Imagine the same day for older and/or disabled people. Note any differ-ences between the two days.

Social welfare law confers few rights on individuals but imposes duties on local authorities to provide or do certain things if specific circumstances are established within a needs framework. Rights are implicit rather than ex-plicit, for example in the local authority's 'duty to assess' for service provi-sion (DPA 1986; NHSCCA 1990); in the health authority's duty to implement, and the local authority's duty to collaborate with, a Care Programme Ap-proach for people referred to specialist psychiatric services (DoH 1990b); and in the joint duty to provide after-care (MHA 1983). Access is to an unspeci-fied service – 'after-care', a 'service plan' or 'assessment of need' – leaving users with little right to force provision of a specific resource. Case law and judicial review decisions have established that local authorities must assess need rationally, provide services for which the 'need' has been established through assessment and meet all and not merely some of the needs identi-fied. However, the passport to 'right' is still 'need', which must be assessed and is thus dependent on professional judgement and discretion. The entitlement is still only to a service rather than to a specific quality of service – 'how' need will be met rather than 'how well'. This discretion may perpetuate stereotypes about appropriate services and result in routinized responses to apparently familiar problems. It may provide help to those in greatest need while overlooking other people's basic rights to choice, warmth, safety and social participation.

Consumerism implies that people have more rights and power than is actually the case. Those rights commonly mentioned have only equivocal support in law and accompanying policy.

Quality of life

The purpose of social care is to maintain and enhance quality of life (DoH 1989a; Centre for Policy on Ageing 1990). The keys are recognizing *personal dignity and value* through respecting and meeting users' needs and wishes; *fulfilment*, through realizing personal aspirations and abilities in all aspects of life; access to services, continuity of provision and opportunities to incur risk, promoting *independence*; and the concept of *privacy* (Social Care Association 1988; DoH 1989c). However, these keys are not rights. When contained in documents issued under section 7 of the Local Authority Social Services Act 1970, they must be followed by local authorities unless good reason can be shown to depart from such guidance. Mainly, however, they are elaborated in documents not issued under this provision. Accordingly, they stand as good practice.

Many people will judge the quality of life to include the right to take reasonable risks and to fail. People with learning difficulties or mental health problems and older people do not have such 'rights'. Their autonomy becomes restricted by notions of welfare and paternalism, focusing on risk, but betraying community anxiety and even rejection. Reasserting these rights becomes, therefore, one objective of social care practice (Ramon 1988; Hugman 1989).

Standard of care

Biehal and Sainsbury (1991) include here: knowing which practitioners are involved, their powers and roles; being listened to; having information about choices; and consenting to intervention where no statutory duty to comply exists. Local authorities must provide information about services but their performance here remains poor (Warburton 1990; SSI 1993e) in terms of accessibility, content, consultation with user groups about information needs, clarity and monitoring effectiveness.

The right to the minimum intervention or least restrictive response possible is codified in regulatory section 7 guidance for children's services (DoH 1989d) but not for social care, demonstrating ambivalence towards quality care. Social care practitioners undertake intimate, complex tasks in working with vulnerable people for which regulation and inspection is essential, yet such oversight as exists may be reduced.

There is no right to a service. Local authorities only have an unequivocal, non-negotiable duty to undertake an assessment when requested by a disabled person or a carer, and enforcing service provision (CSDPA 1970) for assessed needs remains problematic (Norman 1980). No minimum standard of service provision or quality of life has been set. Thus, while social care should include a choice of suitable leisure services and the ability to engage in them (Kitwood and Bredin 1992; Knapp *et al.* 1992), securing a user's presence and participation in the community is difficult. The community does not always want to care. Housing authorities are not required to meet the housing needs of those covered by community care legislation. There is no right to as ordinary a life in as ordinary a home as possible (Arnold *et al.* 1993).

Disabled people remain excluded from anti-discriminatory legislation, and their right to appoint representatives to assist them in negotiations with local authorities (sections 1–3, DPA 1986) remains unimplemented. It has been replaced with guidance that users should be provided with information about advocacy schemes (DoH 1991b). The local authority's legal duty to make fair and unbiased decisions must be contrasted with institutional discrimination against disabled people (Barnes 1992) and policy failure to secure for disabled people a standard of living, and the social and civil rights, comparable with non-disabled people in terms of income, employment, housing, transport and education (Bynoe *et al.* 1991). This effectively excludes disabled people from community activities.

The situation is little better in relation to race, culture, religion and language. Legislation (RRA 1976) requires that local authorities promote equality of opportunity and eliminate discrimination in service provision. However, the NHS and Community Care Act 1990 is silent here and policy guidance, that community care must take account of the circumstances of minority communities and be planned in consultation with them, is not mandatory.

The position in relation to compulsion is complicated. People may only be compulsorily detained in accordance with due procedures. They have a right not to be compelled to accept medication except under particular legal provisions. They have a right to consent to treatment but no right to refuse it. Obstacles exist to securing legal redress when their rights are infringed in the operation of the Mental Health Act 1983. Thus, welfare is not a citizen's right but a privilege delivered differently to different groups by custodians of public resources (Mama 1993).

Participation in social care

Written records, service agreements between users and practitioners, and case reviews are not mandatory requirements. Local authorities may determine how partnership is to be expressed. Users do not have an unequivocal right to attend planning and decision-making meetings, or to be consulted about the closure of residential homes, although some judicial review decisions uphold the local authority's duty to consult. The principle of choice, the opportunity to select independently from a range of options (SSI 1993d), with services supporting the development of ability to choose and to communicate views about issues affecting them (CCETSW 1992a), is undermined by policy guidance which prioritizes resource considerations and professional control, and which views people with learning difficulties and mental health problems not as active citizens, capable of expressing needs and wishes, but as lacking responsibility (Bean and Mounser 1993; Walmsley 1993).

Challenging decisions

Individuals have a right to see social and health care records (APFA 1987; AHRA 1990), although there are restrictions on the range of information open to them (see Braye and Preston-Shoot 1992a). They have the right to express and record disagreement about recorded information. Local authorities are, however, under no duty to publicize this right actively or widely, and the appeals procedure to consider grievances concerning access is likely to favour the local authority, especially when deciding to withhold information on the grounds that release would seriously harm the applicant's physical or mental health.

Social welfare law establishes a right of access to complaints procedures and judicial review of local authority decisions. However, this does not alter the power imbalance between users and providers. To be useful rights and duties must be capable of being enforced. Current procedures are unsatisfactory. First, people are not all equal before the law. Class, gender, race and economic inequalities result in the law reflecting rather than challenging power relationships. Second, unclear drafting of legislation, the discretion given to local authorities regarding the exercise of statutory duties and policy guidance which promotes collective rather than individual recording of unmet need (DoH 1992a) protect local authorities from litigation and accountability.

Third, users must initially use local authority internal complaints procedures. These are biased towards the authority. Unlike in similar procedures established under the Children Act 1989, an independent element is only required when a user requests the review of a previously considered complaint. Those hearing the complaint will not necessarily reflect the gender and racial background of the complainant, who will not necessarily receive adequate support. Users' dependence on services, fears of losing provision if they complain and staff reluctance to endorse positively users' right to complain may all affect use of such procedures (NCC 1993).

Fourth, the requirement (section 50, NHSCCA 1990) to appeal to the Secretary of State to use default powers limits the use of judicial review once the local authority's internal complaints procedure has been exhausted. The judicial review option is further restricted by the initial necessity to seek leave of the court. The criteria for granting leave are unclear, judges demonstrating wide variation in their practice (Dyer 1993). Even when leave is granted, there may be further delays before the case is heard, with individuals less likely than organizations to reach or succeed at final hearing (Dyer 1993). Local authorities not infrequently settle before final hearing, thereby avoiding a review of their decisions.

Fifth, judicial review is not a specific remedy for the complainant. It does not focus on the facts and merits of the situation; nor, if the user succeeds, does it automatically result in the receipt of the service they desire. Rather, a local authority's decisions may be quashed. The process reviews organizational policy and practice for correctness in law and procedure (George 1993).

Sixth, the alternative route of complaint to the Local Commissioner for Administration involves potential time delays. Nor is it a specific remedy for the complainant (Cooper 1990), since the Local Commissioner has no power to enforce recommendations to rectify injustice arising from discrimination, incompetence, delay or other maladministration. Furthermore, in all the possible avenues of complaint, only the individual concerned may seek and establish redress. Rights for user groups are not established by such decisions.

Finally, local authorities have no duty to inform users of these possibilities. The protection provided is also post-event, despite the questions of liberty, risk, compulsion and (ab)use of power potentially involved, although the local authority's complaints procedure can postpone decisions when a complaint is made (DoH 1991g). Procedures should be accessible, quick, impartial and visible, effective and monitored (*Which?* 1993). Of sixteen standards set by the SSI (1993e), only 25 per cent were well met. Local authorities had made good progress in establishing procedures but improvements are necessary concerning timescales, using outcomes to inform service delivery, accessibility and recording.

Towards rights-based practice

Users' rights are uncertain and difficult to enforce when known. Users may remain unaware of local authority duties and powers, and do not always receive appropriate services, such as the Care Programme Approach (Schneider 1993). Adherence to good practice *lessens* the closer one approaches operational reality (Booth *et al.* 1990): agreement on good practice is not necessarily implemented, particularly by those staff most affected. This highlights the importance of enforceable rights for users, coupled with adequate resource levels and training for staff.

The absence of a coherent theory of human need to inform what is or is not acceptable (Doyal and Gough 1991) is accompanied by the absence of a coherent discussion of rights in social care practice. For instance, while the right to confidentiality may be overridden periodically by welfare considerations, a clear articulation and prioritization of basic rights must be accompanied by improved knowledge and skills when, for example, the right to autonomy and choice conflicts with the right of individuals to protection. One consequence is that services provided remain largely determined by custom and convenience, social anxiety, and protective and restrictive attitudes (Norman 1980). Another is the continued absence of an enforceable equal opportunity, anti-discriminatory framework, and of clear guidelines concerning entitlement and levels of service. A third consequence is the continuation of existing power relationships, which ensure both an unfair distribution of resources, with attendant social and moral costs of inequitable treatment, frustration and internalized oppression (Galligan 1992), and inequitable access to means of attaining rights and securing the performance of local authority duties.

An alternative is a rights-based approach to meeting basic needs, where rights are protections to secure and prioritize essential and valued aspects of human nature and social relations (Freeden 1991) and where needs fundamental to citizenship are defined. The basic needs of survival and autonomy are the same for all groups (Doyal and Gough 1991). Survival means resources to promote and maintain physical and mental health. Personal autonomy means the capacity to initiate active citizenship and social participation. This depends on access to knowledge and on opportunities for action. This requires that social constraints on such action are minimized, whether these are external to individuals or intrapersonal, internalized oppression arising from experiences of powerlessness (Barber 1991). Personal autonomy includes the ability to question and criticize, and opportunities to participate in agreeing or changing normative structures. Thus, services are a means to an end rather than an end in themselves. Satisfiers of these basic needs will vary, dependent on power structures, access to resources and the individual's position in society. Accordingly, individuals and groups must have the right to define their needs and possible satisfiers of them, together with the power to achieve this through access to resources to ensure that existing power relations do not exclude people from their rights.

Such a model adopts a three-dimensional power relationship, engaging not only with the individual but also with the political and structural context within which her or his needs will be met. Consumerism and existing service provision ignore the reality of power (Taylor 1989), especially the impact of class, age, gender and race on access to opportunities to define needs and satisfiers. In the three-dimensional model, individuals have the right to define their own needs, and the rights necessary for the realization of meaningful citizenship (Barton 1993). These must include not only privacy, dignity, independence, choice, fulfilment, community presence and participation, competence and partnership (SSI 1993b, d); not only access to information and complaints procedures, written agreements and an absence of bias; but also the right to optimal social care provision (Doyal 1993), defined from user and worker experience and expertise, and the rights to treatment for physical and mental ill-health and to adequate resources to maintain and maximize well-being.

In the standardized exercise of local authority powers and duties, survival and autonomy may be undermined. The origin of user-advocacy and self-directed work (Mullender and Ward 1991) lies in the disempowering nature of much service delivery, its failure to promote social participation and critical autonomy. A rights-based approach prioritizes a more equal, rather than a more acceptably unequal, society (Barton 1993).

Resources

Promoting health and autonomy and preventing serious harm requires *resources*. The cost-effective use of resources has become a dominant imperative in service provision (Audit Commission 1986). The objective of assessment is to provide the right level of intervention and support to help people achieve the maximum independence possible and their full potential *within available resources* (DoH 1989a). Good practice provisions (DoH 1993d) need only be implemented 'as resources permit'. The decision whether people referred to specialist psychiatric services can be treated realistically in the community will be taken by professionals in the light of available resources (DoH 1990b). Clearly inpatient treatment, or residential care, will be offered if needs cannot be met from available resources, even if on other criteria such provision is inappropriate. What message does this send to people already vulnerable or disadvantaged by age, disability or illness?

The meaning of cost-effective use of resources, of value for money, remains ambiguous. Should, for example, individuals in need be given resources to meet their needs when the cost of such provision is disproportionate to the benefit (likely to be) derived (Levick 1992)? Is prioritizing those in greatest need (DoH 1989a) cost-effective, or should greater investment be made in preventive services? Using community care finance to provide intensive, preventive support may meet needs and promote rights, following the principle of normalization. However, resource scarcity may prompt decisions based on other imperatives.

To juxtapose without comment requirements for services to be user-focused, to involve users in deciding how services might satisfy their needs, with demands to 'live' within available resources and obscure levels of unmet need by recording wishes (DoH 1992a) is to engage in a con trick. Outcome objectives of improved quality of life and improved resource distribution are not necessarily compatible (Huxley 1993). Quality can be measured by adequacy: level and volume of service; accessibility; competence of service delivered; efficiency in resource use; relevance for users (DoH 1992b). These measures are not necessarily compatible. Moreover, users' voices are likely to become lost if practitioners, managers and politicians by-pass political and moral questions by imposing and accepting a rationing, gatekeeping role. The issue ultimately is not whether but how resources should be prioritized, and the absence of explicit criteria should be openly debated and negotiated (Ellis 1993). The confidence trick is to pretend that such debates are unnecessary.

One outcome is that practitioners prioritize and ration services locally, while being urged (BASW 1990) not to collude with the imposition of hardship because of society's failure to make appropriate provision, or to compromise their professional values and practice by failing to assess honestly and openly vulnerable people's needs because of the spectre of legal challenges arising from unmet assessed needs. A second outcome is that resource-driven definitions of need and quality ignore structural inequalities, thereby exacerbating power imbalances. The third outcome is the loss of service innovation. The crisis rather than preventive approach into which resource constrained agencies become trapped results in standardized provision. It is naive to suppose that needs-led assessments remain unaffected by knowledge of resource availability, whatever the purchaser–provider split. Barclay (1982) found evidence that workers identified fewer problems than users.

The permissive and fragmented nature of adult services legislation has meant that resource availability has traditionally influenced levels of service provision. Clear duties do exist, to provide an assessment (section 4, DPA 1986) and after-care (section 117, MHA 1983), but more often duties arise once local authorities have agreed a need for services. Otherwise, local authorities have powers to promote the welfare of older and/or disabled people, and to provide preventive, care and after-care services to people with physical and mental illness. Services are at the dual mercy of financial constraints and local definitions of need, and additionally of the interaction between them. Services are often, therefore, inappropriate to the needs of particular individuals (Baldwin 1986; Humphries 1992; Smale *et al.* 1993), for instance in terms of race and culture, because situations are only seen in professional terms.

Contrast this position with the argument that people should have a right to optimal satisfaction of basic needs, and a right to participate in deciding how such satisfaction should occur in practice (Doyal and Gough 1991). Optimal satisfaction here equates to the best available, which, when this outstretches available resources, is replaced with a constrained optimum which specifies the highest level of satisfaction possible. Need prioritized as a mandate would involve:

- services based on users' felt and expressed needs except where statutory duties of protection operate owing to assessed risk, with practitioners seeking to understand users' lived experience;
- definition of common human needs, such as warmth, housing, education and safety, which are then addressed by policy and practice, to enable people to achieve and maintain physical health, autonomy and social participation;
- routine use of advocacy, to enable more effective questioning of assessments and services of which care managers and providers are a part, to provide information about resources and possibilities, and to challenge internalized oppression where users may have lower expectations of services and define their needs accordingly.

Theme 2: who is competent to make what decisions?

The second major challenge in social care is the question of who makes decisions about people's lives, and by reference to what values.

> People should have *autonomy* in the decisions they make about their lives.
>
> Sometimes people do not make sound decisions and may need *protection* from harm, or others need protection from them.
>
> Sometimes people need help *to take control* over decisions about their lives.

All three statements may be deduced from the values implicit in legislation on decision-making, and in social care practice.

Autonomy

Exercise 4.4.   For what reasons, by what mechanisms and with what protections do you believe people may be disqualified from making their own decisions?

At a simplistic level the law upholds individual autonomy in decision-making. The common law test of capacity sets a low threshold of under-standing. In most circumstances competence and rationality are presumed; the quality of the decision is irrelevant.

The autonomy position has been colonized by those advocating choice for service users within an ideology of consumerism, and is linked to debates about quality by the assumption (DoH 1989a, 1990a, 1991e) that it is regulated by consumer choice within a free and competitive market. Choice is viewed as central to assisting people to fuller independence and dignity. However, this emphasis has not reduced the level of professional control. Users do not control their own budgets to purchase what they require. Choice is further restricted by a fixed menu of services (Flynn and Hurley 1993a, b) which provide providers with stability over time but limit flexibility of spot purchasing. However, policy equivocation about choice is revealed most clearly by the acknowledgement (SSI 1993b) of constraints imposed on social services departments by limited resources, of the inevitability of limited life options experienced by disabled people and of their limited numbers (that is low cost) and experience justifying efforts to afford greater choice. Put another way, resources and paternalism, not autonomy and rights, underpin this view of choice.

This notion of autonomy is more restrictive than the critical version envisaged by Doyal and Gough (1991). Effectively, it leaves structural inequalities unaltered and leaves open the possibility of abuse of power. Providing information and some participation in decision-making is a very different vision from providing resources and enhancing people's skills to enable them, individually and collectively, both to develop personally and also to challenge unequal access to resources, which limits genuine autonomy (Atkinson 1991), and the normative judgements on which professional and agency decisions have previously been based. Consumerism assumes that people have an equal ability to enforce their rights, to participate in decision-making and to control their own lives. Social care's commitment to autonomy is founded on longstanding notions of self-determination which have more recently developed to accommodate a commitment to challenging inequality of access to *opportunity* for self-determination. As such, social care would challenge the notions embedded within consumerism.

Protection

Legislation sometimes disqualifies people from decision-making competency, justifying intervention by others in the interests of people's *welfare* or as *protective* of their own or someone else's interests. The Mental Health Act 1983, for example, while partly designed to protect vulnerable people's rights, provides for the deprivation of liberty and compulsory psychiatric treatment in the interests of the health or safety of the person concerned or for the protection of others. A parallel common law regime for treatment other than for mental disorder exists, and for people not compulsorily detained but incapable of consenting. It is similarly dominated by professional paternalism (Fennell 1990) and justifies, by reference to 'best interests' and 'welfare', extensive powers to control behaviour in such sensitive and personal arenas as abortion and sterilization. The control of sexuality (SOA 1956) raises considerable dilemmas for social care practice. Whether originally conceived as a means of protecting people with learning disability from sexual exploitation, or of controlling their reproduction, legislation effectively makes it impossible for a woman with severe learning disability to consent to sexual intercourse. Professionals wishing to promote the rights of people with learning disabilities to engage in sexual relationships potentially act outside a legally permitted context (Gunn 1991) in an area where legislation impedes the development of ethical practice and encourages a professional response which infantilizes and assumes the need to protect people rather than to learn from their resourcefulness and enable them to make informed choices about sexual behaviour (McCarthy and Thompson 1991).

To assume, of course, that paternalism is automatically bad and autonomy good is simplistic (Darbyshire 1991). An ethical duty of care will sometimes require practitioners to minimize harm, to prioritize welfare above self-determination. People's competency may vary, affected by health-related issues and/or different levels of complexity and decision required (Atkinson 1991). However, as the predominant use of section 47 of the NAA 1948 with older people illustrates, risk and autonomy are tolerated differently for different groups.

Society is inconsistent in the risks it allows (Norman 1980). For some groups attitudes demonstrate paternalistic over-protection from risk rather than an acknowledgement of the right to self-determination. Norman concludes that practitioners require better tools for assessing risks and strengths, although she compromises this call for improved decision-making by locating it within available resources rather than arguing for optimal need satisfaction. Arguably, practice in relation to risk has not always distinguished between protection and excessive or intrusive intervention; between enhancing an individual's capacity for self-direction and independence, and acting when protection is necessary; between different options to improve quality of life. Thus, in social care, assessments have sometimes been incremental and reactive; new information not considered alongside previous knowledge; patterns of risk and needs not collated into a comprehensive whole (SSI 1993b). Admission to residential care has been based on whim, chance and absence of choice (Sinclair et al. 1988; Bywaters 1991) rather than assessment of risk and the use of residential options within flexible and responsive services.

Assessing risk is rendered more difficult by the absence of effective legal frameworks to protect adults from abuse and neglect, and by the not infrequent absence of harm-free or risk-free options (Carson 1988), with the result that practitioners are confronted with dilemma management. Assessing risk is complicated further by the essential unknowability of situations and fears of negative publicity. There are no reliable indicators or predictors of risk; neither can all the variables be controlled. Indeed, to try is likely to result in oppressive or defensive practice. Some risk or uncertainty must be tolerated. How much has not been debated in relation to social care practice.

Empowering practice suggests that practitioners should assume competency rather than incapacity, and recognize that lack of opportunities rather than capacity may create difficulties or restrict choices for individuals (Day 1987). This requires a strict test of incapacity, perhaps sustained lack of capacity for intellectual understanding, consistent reasoning, confidence to interact and recognition of responsibility for action (Doyal 1993); or inability to understand information in simple terms relevant to a decision, including information about reasonably foreseeable consequences of taking or failing to take the decision, or to retain the information long enough to take an effective decision (Law Commission 1993).

A clear definition should be accompanied by codified procedures which protect users' rights, with concern for welfare activated only in those areas where capacity to act responsibly is severely diminished (Fairbairn 1987). A strict test of capacity may require practice shifts in social care, with practitioners having to be competent in allowing users to take risks when these are fully understood (Biggs and Weinstein 1991). Anti-oppressive practice would respect users' expressed wishes and needs (Stevenson and Parsloe 1993) and assert individuals' right to take risks, even where these are not fully understood, except where serious risk of harm exists. The worker's role is to share and facilitate access to, but not impose, information, knowledge, definitions and expertise; to share concerns and agree objectives. This may involve addressing internalized oppression since competence may be affected by what individuals believe they may or can (safely) do. It means moving away from an expert model towards one of mutual education, concerned to maximize users' abilities, individually and collectively, to define issues which concern them and identify appropriate action.

It follows that practitioners must specify what knowledge, information and reasons are used to justify protective intervention or an assessment of incapacity. A key skill is, therefore, the effective gathering, recording and analysis of information to determine the level of intervention necessary to safeguard and promote welfare. This, in turn, depends on practitioners evaluating the effect on practice of personally held images of 'acceptable' behaviour and risks, scrutinizing their practice for cultural, sexist, able-bodied and/ or ageist assumptions, and questioning the influence on their decisions of anxiety or prevailing professional ideologies and cultures (Braye and Preston-Shoot 1992a). It depends too on a model of decision-making which distinguishes different types of risks, evaluates hazards, dangers and their likelihood, and considers in partnership with users and carers (Kitwood and Bredin 1992; Knapp *et al.* 1992) the available courses of action and their likely outcomes (Brearley 1982; Braye and Preston-Shoot 1992a).

Such practice must be underpinned by an organizational response, particularly in the form of statements in community care plans and procedural guidelines about practice aims, and the types and degrees of autonomy and informed risk-taking which will be supported, together with structures to enable practitioners to manage such practice (see Chapter 8).

Partnership and empowerment

In this third dimension of the mandate, state intervention is justified by reference to principles of partnership and empowerment where the aim is

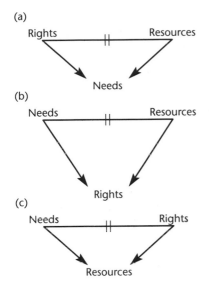

(a)

In a situation where resources are insufficient to meet the demands people might make if they exercise rights, the concept of need is useful as a mediator to assist rationing.

(b)

Where need is greater than can be resourced, the concept of rights is useful because people do not have a right to have their needs met, or a hierarchy of eligibility can be established where some have more right than others.

(c)

Where people do not have a right to what they need, and perhaps do not need what they have a right to, the concept of resources is a useful mediator – people are given what can be afforded.

Figure 4.1 Triangulation of needs, rights and resources.
Source: Braye and Preston-Shoot (1994).

not to control but to facilitate and promote self-determination. Chapters 2 and 5 analyse these principles more fully. They are used extensively in policy guidance and are meant to permeate all interactions between users, carers and providers (DoH 1991b). However, as envisaged here the power remains with the professionals, while user groups and welfare professionals have developed the concepts to challenge the oppression which undermines people's autonomy and choices, and professional ownership of the power to define issues and prescribe solutions. This moves the focus beyond the procedural relationship between local authorities and users.

Triangles

Deciding who should have access to what services is made much more complex by the way in which needs, rights and resources exist in dynamic tension with each other, often pulling in different directions. Their relationship may be seen as one of triangulation, a process whereby the conflict between two mandates is by-passed by a third. Any combination is possible, thus keeping all three mandates alive (Braye and Preston-Shoot 1994) – see Figure 4.1.

In determining who should make decisions, based on what values, the tension between the three mandates of autonomy, protection and empowerment again leads to triangulation between them – see Figure 4.2.

The covert alliance between two conflictual concepts is detoured through a third. Such interactions help to explain why the intricate balance of the relationship remains predominantly stable despite its conflicts. In apparently

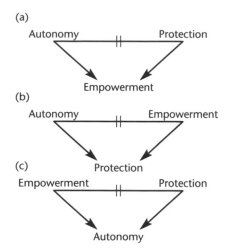

(a)

Autonomy ———————— Protection

Empowerment

If people do what they want, they may place themselves at risk, so we must help them make good decisions in whatever areas they can.

(b)

Autonomy ———————— Empowerment

Protection

If we intervene in people's lives, that limits their autonomy, but it is justified in their own interests.

(c)

Empowerment ———————— Protection

Autonomy

Empowerment and protection get very mixed up – it is often difficult to tell the difference, so we will respect people's wishes and choices.

Figure 4.2 Triangulation of autonomy, protection and empowerment.
Source: Braye and Preston-Shoot (1994).

'solving' the problem, such processes enable avoidance of a debate that would bring more fundamental resolution by answering the question of which mandate has priority.

The source of the tensions partly lies in the relationships between those who are stakeholders in social care. The Department of Health translates government intentions and legal mandates into policy and practice guidance, and has a controlling and regulatory interest which reflects dominant political ideology. Social services departments carry the complex influences of statute, finance, professionalism and service user opinion, together with local political mandates and accountability. Service users bring an individual interest in how legal mandates are interpreted, and a growing collective voice in seeking to influence what services are offered and how statutory power is used.

What will bring about change? Seeking clarity about the purposes of policy and practice will involve prioritization of conflicting imperatives: that needs and rights notwithstanding, resources must prevail; or that resource availability and need assessment must defer to rights. Where purposes do not overlap but demonstrate potential for divergence and conflict, or where practitioners are unable or unwilling to prioritize because of equally balanced competing demands or unease about how prioritization is determined, this must be debated between professionals, users, advocacy groups, agencies and politicians. This higher-level discourse would openly address eight key questions:

1 How should practitioners manage accountability to employers, government, users and professional values?
2 How should conflicts between social care policy and professional values be resolved?

3 What is a professional ethical duty of care?
4 How should welfare be interpreted? If avoidance of risk, how is this best achieved? If intervention when a person's capacity to act responsibly is diminished, how is such capacity to be understood?
5 What rights should users and carers have?
6 What level of risk is appropriate? When is control appropriate?
7 How should people's basic needs, for survival and autonomy, be met and to what level?
8 What is the best way in which the state and its citizens can work together to ensure the optimal satisfaction of needs?

5 Power, partnership and empowerment

Partnership and empowerment are key features in both policy language and the values talk that surrounds social care. Chapter 2 began to explore their meaning, identifying their location in the traditional and radical value bases respectively. What unites them is their concern with power: with how professionals use their power, and additionally with wider power relationships in society and their impact on the lives of those who use services.

The reasons for the concern with power are complex and contradictory, reflecting the interaction of several influences. First, awareness has grown that services are provided in ways which at best are inappropriate to people's needs, and at worst collude with and perpetuate inequalities. Statutory services have failed to offer black communities appropriate services, leaving them on the periphery of social care (Jones *et al.* 1992). The services provided have been founded on a deficit model (Macdonald 1991), focusing on problems and weakness, and characterized by negative cultural stereotyping, assumptions of individual pathology and an inadequate knowledge base (B. Ahmad 1990). The dominance of white Eurocentric thinking in service provision has spawned two damaging approaches (Dominelli 1988). *Assimilationist* thinking has assumed that services provided are basically sound and that black people can take advantage of them if they wish. This 'colour blind' approach, treating everyone as the same, reflects an investment in preserving the assumed cultural homogeneity of British society (Naik 1991). *Cultural pluralism* requires services to be sensitive to cultural diversity and respond to people's 'special needs' on dimensions such as language, diet and religion. It assumes that Britain is a white society to which other groups have been appended, whose cultural characteristics can be tolerated provided they are construed as different from a white norm (Naik 1993). It is a superficial and paternalistic response (Husband 1991), which in a context of race equality is fair and appropriate but in the context of racism effectively deconstructs black resistance (Sivanandan 1991). Based on cultural stereotyping and pathologizing, it fails to amend the ideology of white superiority that is an essential feature of racism (OSDC 1991).

Social care services are thus part of a framework of institutionalized racism, a view reinforced by the over-representation of black people in measures which exert social control (compulsory mental health admissions, criminal justice procedures) and under-representation in supportive, facilitative service provision. That this has been known for some time, and yet not acted on by statutory agencies (Butt *et al.* 1991), further illustrates the power of the dominant ideology.

Feminist thinking (Dominelli and McLeod 1989) has contributed a perspective which tackles the innumerable ways in which patriarchal social relations undermine women's well-being, and locates the origin of women's social problems in social factors, not women's psyche. Recognition of gender oppression, and challenge to both the definition of and solutions to problems based on it, are essential spheres of activity, together with both collective action and individualized responses which demonstrate the negative impact of statutory social care provision on women in their roles as carers, users and workers.

Mental health service users have also demanded changes to services, dominated as they have been by reliance on institutional care, pharmocological treatment and professional power. Survivors have experienced oppression arising from the perceived quality, range and relevance of services (Survivors Speak Out 1986; Rogers *et al.* 1993), the failure to protect from institutional discrimination (Bynoe *et al.* 1991) and psychiatry's recruitment to the task of social control (Sashidharan 1989; Fernando 1991; Ussher 1991). The complex interaction of various forms of discrimination ensures that many who experience the negative consequences of labelling and stigma on mental health grounds will have additional forms of oppression, such as racism, sexism and homophobia, to contend with.

Common demands have been: the right to be treated as people not 'cases'; rights to information about and choices in treatment; access to safe environments; recognition that distress has a wide range of meanings over and above that implied by psychiatric diagnosis, and that people in distress need housing, money and refuge rather than psychotropic drugs (Wallcraft 1993). Users and survivors have: demanded a reappraisal of the value base of service provision (Lawson 1991); developed guidelines for an empowering service (Read and Wallcraft 1992), including changes to the dehumanizing and depersonalizing experience of hospital care (GPMH and Camden Consortium 1988); set out the agenda for user control of services (Chamberlin 1988), community care structures (Beeforth *et al.* 1990) and mechanisms of participation (NHSTD 1993); campaigned for services which respond more appropriately to women's distress and do not expose them to further abuse (Women in Mind 1986; Gorman 1992); and contributed to an understanding of how services must respond to racial diversity (Webb-Johnson 1991). Protest against the medicalization of distress has resulted in the creation of alternative, more relevant networks for responding to and helping people manage distress, user-led networks which operate outside statutory systems, attempting to compensate for the perceived deficiencies of those services.

Involved here is a reappraisal of the traditional power balance between users and professionals, a demand that providers hear and respond to what is wanted rather than impose non-negotiated and often oppressive solutions. Empowerment happens not just because powerful people give away power, but because oppressed people engage in wresting it from them, speaking out *against* abuse and oppression, and *for* changes in systems, demanding a radical rather than a liberal or functionalist form of partnership (Adams 1990), which alters rather than works within existing power relations and traditional definitions of need and agency responsibilities. The mandate from users imposes a dual responsibility: that services should be *non-oppressive* – should neither negatively stereotype vulnerability through age, disability or mental health, nor oppress people through their race, sex, sexuality or class status – and that practitioners must be *anti-oppressive* in how they engage with users and their networks in challenging oppressive practice and experienced oppression.

Second, professional concern about structural inequality and the unequal relationship between users and practitioners, together with the realization that what practitioners think people need is frequently not what users say they want, has resulted in an emphasis on user involvement in assessment, decision-making and contract-based work (Corden and Preston-Shoot 1987), and explicit consideration of differences of opinion and of the power dynamics between those involved. The growing professional emphasis on anti-oppressive practice requires practitioners to be aware of how stereotypical images of people affect assumptions about their competence, and thus their rights and autonomy. It requires that structural issues and social change goals are incorporated alongside individually focused work. Services which fail to engage with issues of race, gender, disability, sexuality, age and poverty, and which are managed from a white, middle-class, usually male and able-bodied outlook, will at best lack important perspectives because they neither identify nor use the diversity of people's experiences, strengths and skills. At worst they are oppressive because they presume targets and purposes of intervention, and omit questions of rights, equality and social justice.

Attention focuses on how professionals use and abuse the power of their position: exerting control along three dimensions by taking active measures to prevent users occupying influential and authoritative positions; failing to act to remove barriers and obstacles to participation; and/or creating a reality in which it is normal for users to be passive and quiescent (Drake 1992). Even mechanisms developed from an ethos of power sharing and negotiation, such as written agreements, are abused when used to impose prescriptions, professional agendas and control (Nelken 1987, 1989).

There are two broad strands in the professional abuse of power (Wardhaugh and Wilding 1993): misguided pursuit of acceptable policy goals; and gratuitous actions unrelated to any legitimate policy aim. Key factors associated with abuse of power include the value position that is taken concerning service users, whereby people devalued by society are placed beyond the bounds of moral obligation, and the degree of powerlessness and isolation experienced by staff.

A third mandate for empowerment and partnership is legislative (NHSCCA 1990) or, more specifically, derived from associated policy guidance. The ideology here, however, is quite different. Power in this context means consumer power, the power to purchase, seen as an essential component in creating a market economy of welfare. Quality of service is regulated and improved by users' freedom of choice to buy or not to buy. Working in partnership here means facilitating users' expression of choice. The mechanisms required are access to information, decision-making procedures and channels of complaint; negotiation; and involvement in assessment and planning. Even here partnership and empowerment are difficult to achieve (SSI 1993b, e). The government-initiated Users and Carers Group, established to monitor community care implementation, has encountered numerous official barriers to participation (Beresford 1994).

Given these influential mandates, and noting that greater user involvement was advocated several decades ago (Seebohm Report 1968), it is important to explore why the thought does not guarantee the deed, why practising partnership and empowerment is not that simple.

First, the mandate from welfare law does not unequivocally embrace the concept of partnership. As discussed in Chapter 4, legislation and policy guidance continue to promote professionally defined concepts of 'need' and 'care' rather than rights, and fail to endorse user-led assessment by the emphasis given to cost-effectiveness and resource availability, and by the power given to professionals (DoH 1991b). Similarly, consensus between those exercising choice is assumed. Guidance blandly refers to users and carers in one breath, with little recognition of how views may differ, or be influenced by interpersonal dynamics. In reality, conflict is not unusual between users and their families, the perspectives of carers under pressure resulting in quite different choices from those of the person being cared for.

Community care reforms have left traditional power balances relatively intact. Services must take into account the needs and circumstances of minority communities, and be planned in consultation with them (DoH 1989a, 1990a), but local authorities may determine the form of consultation undertaken, and their track-record in developing racially appropriate services is unimpressive (Dutt 1990). The key targets of accessibility, appropriateness, adequacy and accountability derive from white European norms and reflect stereotypical images of family roles in relation to caring. Additionally, emphasis on cost-effectiveness encourages economies of scale which inevitably address the needs of majority groups rather than providing the individualized flexibility required to cater for diverse communities (Mirza 1991).

Both ring-fenced money for services through MISG and access to care programme planning for individuals are targeted at people in contact with formal psychiatric services, despite survivors' criticism of these services. While opportunities must be provided for patients to take part in decisions about their proposed care programmes, to discuss different treatment possibilities and agree the programmes to be implemented (DoH 1990b), the range of services upon which these possibilities are based still does not reflect planned, systematic and empowering consultation with users (DoH 1993a).

This legal ambivalence reflects the different and sometimes discriminatory purposes for which society uses the law: promoting rights while preserving power structures, sanctioning risk and autonomy while retaining social control (Braye and Preston-Shoot 1992a). Even where legislation does exist to promote equality of opportunity (section 71, RRA 1976), provisions are so vague and sanctions so weak that the law has little impact. Given that legislators reflect a dominant ethnic, gender, racial and class configuration, it is unsurprising that legislation influences the dynamics of dominance and subordination, and lends itself to being recruited by powerful groups for purposes of preserving power structures and controlling those who threaten them (Braye and Preston-Shoot 1993b).

Social care practice too is in a muddle about empowerment and partnership. Professional practice espouses a radical, anti-oppressive agenda where partnership is user-directed and challenges traditional power relationships, while continuing to render oppression invisible by privatizing public ills or, if challenging unfairness, doing so within a professionally led agenda and existing power structures (Phillipson 1992). As long as partnership and empowerment remain undefined in legislation, differing interpretations are possible. Partnership is used to describe anything from token consultation to a total devolution of power and control. Additionally, it is meant to bring some magic ingredient to the relationship between users and providers: to benefit people by bringing their unique perspective into the bargaining situation and thus improving the quality of decisions made; users' knowledge and experience is also held to give them the ability and motivation to represent others in similar situations (Newman 1993). Similar confusions surround empowerment (see Chapter 2), used to describe the rights, choices and control demanded by the self-advocacy movement and the mechanisms of consumerism prescribed in policy guidance.

Emerging professional principles for partnership practice (Marsh and Fisher 1992) promote user choice without clarifying how professionally led consumerism empowers users, and argue that statutory mandates can form the basis of partnership without addressing the criticism that this is not partnership but participation in a preset agenda. In the context of multiple partnerships with users, carers and professional networks, to whom practitioners owe primary allegiance remains unclear when parties disagree or authorities fail to implement their statutory duties.

The conflicts in the system are denied, with empowerment and partnership recruited to detour conflicts between different stakeholders in the welfare system. Figure 5.1 illustrates how discussion about the imbalance of power between professionals and service users is avoided through assumed consensus about partnership and empowerment, which may have different meanings for those involved but with which no one can disagree. Fears and anxieties are defended against, the concepts helping everyone to feel better. Figure 5.2 demonstrates how tensions and conflicts which originate between two parties are played out elsewhere, a third party regulating the relationship between two others (Byng-Hall 1980) and thereby assuaging anxiety and

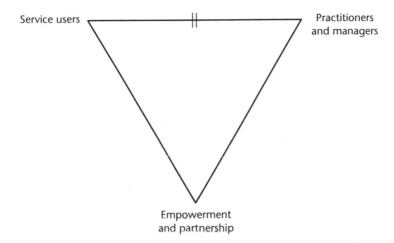

Figure 5.1   Denial of conflicts between professionals and service users.
Source: Braye and Preston-Shoot (1993b).

satisfying needs. In Figure 5.2a the core tension is between government and social welfare, the dialogue about the nature of power and inequality and the role of welfare professions. Users are invited by government to join an anti-professional position, enticed by the prospect of talking direct to policy-makers. The professionals hold out the prospect of 'true partnership' leading to better quality services, in return for which users must not rock the boat.

In Figure 5.2b the core tension is between the state and its citizens, the dialogue about rights, needs and citizenship. Social welfare is recruited by the state to provide services for needy people to obscure questions of rights, in return for resources and legitimacy. Users recruit social welfare to the task of meeting need, to which professionals respond in return for demand remaining at a reasonable, affordable level. In Figure 5.2c the core tension is between welfare professions and users, the dialogue about professional power. Users invite government to intervene when professionals are experienced as oppressive. Social care relies on its statutory mandate to justify its actions, in return for continued endorsement of its existence.

The triangulated nature of this system is not addressed because it protects the parties from feared calamities: for government, of opening the floodgates of need; for social welfare professions, of losing their autonomy; for users, of losing services. Solutions are repeated in revised and more elaborate forms, while assumptions, beliefs and fears are not articulated (Preston-Shoot and Agass 1990). Within such collusions, particularly between the state and professional groups, values are eroded (Borsay 1986; Cornwell 1992/3) and their impact on practice is minimized.

What, then, will bring about change and ensure that the value base of empowerment is strongly articulated in social care practice? The three key components follow.

(a)

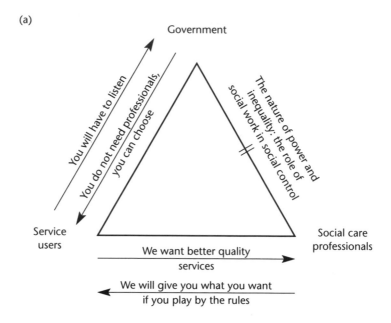

(b)

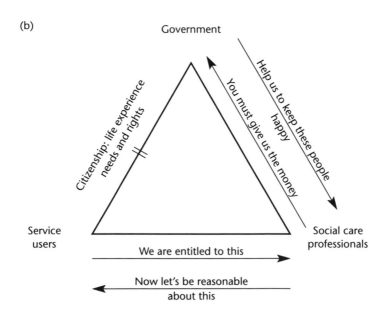

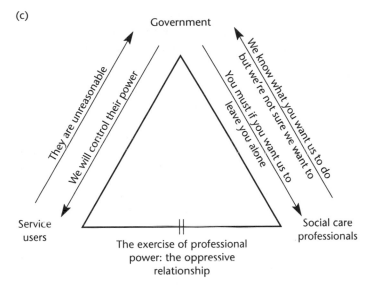

Figure 5.2 Triangulation of government, users and professionals.
Source: Braye and Preston-Shoot (1993b).

The conceptual frame

A conceptual frame for empowering practice contains two core ingredients.

Power

The first ingredient is the acknowledgement of power and its operation within societal structures, social relations and personal relationships. Inequalities of power and status are embedded into people's consciousness and social structures (Frosh 1987). The terms 'user' and 'professional' conjure up images of 'appropriate' behaviour, where the power of expectations and reward encourage people to act in character. Changing power relationships requires the identification of sources of power, and how the elements involved interact together to produce a 'fit'. Consideration must be given to whether power is imposed or conferred, and thus whether it can be given away or must be taken. Each is possible.

There is the power to reward, legitimate, coerce or punish (French and Raven 1959), strongly equated with positional, organizational and statutory authority, and with status derived from gender, class and race (Payne and Scott 1982). Power derived from knowledge and expertise connects with sapiential authority, which comes from experience, training, information and resources. Referent power, deriving from charisma and willingness by others to refer or defer to individuals, relates to authority of relevance, which is assigned by virtue of knowledge possessed or seen as relevant to the situation. The use of referent power is likely to elicit identification; of positional power, compliance; of sapiential power, internalization.

Professionals thus have access to considerable power *over* others: to define issues, allow access to resources and carry out key tasks conferred by the state (Hugman 1991). Social care provision, therefore, is one vehicle through which dominant beliefs are transmitted, and easily becomes normalizing and repressive, recruited to the task of preserving power structures rooted in inequality. Mental health professionals, for example, carry the power to control and contain distress, to apply a chemical or legal straitjacket on behaviour that is inconvenient, bizarre, frightening or upsetting. Woven into the operation of mentalism, or sane chauvinism (Chamberlin 1988), can be observed the additional influences of institutionalized racism and sexism, which lend these powers to the maintaining of control of specific groups of people – black women and men, black and white women – whose 'difference' or 'protest' is threatening and must be silenced, or whose distressed responses to oppression are medicalized and treated, leaving the behaviour of the oppressors unaddressed.

Along with recognition of sources of professional power comes the necessity of conceptually locating users in their class, race, gender and community context, and acknowledging the politics that define their status (Husband 1991). Important here is an integrated perspective on the oppressions experienced by people as a result of social divisions and the institutionalized patterns of dominance and subordination that characterize social relations. This means recognizing that the experience of oppression is complex, that within broad divisions of race, gender, class, age, (dis)ability, sexuality and health status are subtle constellations of similarity and difference which unite and separate people. Older women's experience, for instance, of the oppressive impact of capitalism, ageism and patriarchal society is mediated through race, class, disability, sexuality, age and a range of other factors which combine in unique personal histories (Hughes and Mtezuka 1992). The impact of being black in a racist society similarly has a significance that is affected and compounded by gender, sexuality, age and class.

In deconstructing the notion of oppression based on broad, simple groupings there are dangers: of detracting from the power of collective resistance, and of failing to recognize the enduring, pervasive and inescapable oppression experienced by black people. Recognition of heterogeneity, however, offers considerably more potential, particularly at the level of individual practice, for understanding and helping to empower people on dimensions which are significant and important for them as individuals, and in ways which recognize the dynamics of power between individual professionals and users engaged in that encounter. Such an 'audit' of power, in terms of all parties to a service provision relationship, offers an overview of the raw materials of empowerment, of the dimensions on which power is, or is potentially, abused, and of the sources and resources for change and enhanced positive control.

Anti-discriminatory or anti-oppressive practice

The second core ingredient of a conceptual frame is an understanding of the scope of empowerment and, based on that understanding, the exercise of choice about the focus of activity. A key concept here is the distinction between one-, two- and three-dimensional power relationships (Rees 1991) (see Chapter 4). These indicate choices for practitioners about who controls the agenda, how power is used and whether the political context is explored explicitly. The labels anti-discriminatory practice and anti-oppressive practice are often used interchangeably, but they differ in important respects. The former is reformist, challenging unfairness or inequity in how services are delivered or removing barriers to access. It links with a two-dimensional use of power which seeks change, but within officially sanctioned rules, procedures and structures. Anti-oppressive practice is more radical, seeking a fundamental change in power structures and exploitative relationships which maintain inequality and oppression (Phillipson 1992). Its use of power is three-dimensional since it acknowledges structural inequality and exploitative legal, social and economic relationships, and seeks a fundamental realignment of power relationships in the wider social context.

Anti-discriminatory practice would ensure that consultation with users occurs, both about levels and types of provision and about individual needs and preferences. This practice is envisaged by social care policy guidance. Workers will additionally work to ensure that services are not biased in their suitability for, say, black users, that resources are shared equally and that compulsory powers are not used differentially in respect of different communities. It respects a medical model of distress, disability or ageing, integrating psychological stress perspectives and encompassing psychosocial intervention techniques. Anti-oppressive social care practice, however, involves active pressure for changes in resource provision to ensure the wider range and choice of services required but not yet provided. It promotes user-led and controlled initiatives, and campaigns to change oppressive legal structures and practices. It challenges individualized, medical models of need, admitting the possibility of alternative social construct models of disability or ageing, acknowledging the complex factors which contribute to users' experiences and the political purposes of society's responses.

Anti-discriminatory practice, at least in relation to some issues concerning racism and sexism, is supported by the legal framework. Anti-oppressive practice is not. Yet it is this approach which will enable workers and users to identify how power is exercised and experienced, to acquire the confidence to address exclusion and powerlessness, to address the personal and interpersonal impact of structural inequalities and social constructions, and to ensure that practice does not mirror or reinforce present power imbalances. Neither anti-discriminatory nor anti-oppressive practice equate with the one-dimensional use of power, where workers control the agenda and demand compliance. Yet such practice is not unfamiliar. It is easier for everyone if 'mad' people take their medication, can be forced to do so if they refuse, and are grateful for the services provided to contain distress so that it does not trouble or cause society to change.

Figure 5.3 demonstrates some of the differences between anti-discriminatory and anti-oppressive practice. Partnership holds a curious position within this framework. Partnership (see Chapter 2) is used to describe differing practices and, accordingly, is best conceived of as a continuum (Pugh and De'Ath 1989) from involvement in and consultation about decision-making processes

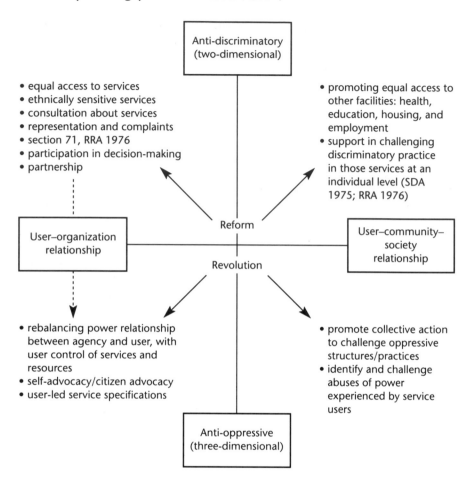

Figure 5.3 Anti-discriminatory and anti-oppressive practice.

within predetermined limits, through collaboration in defining issues and options, and beyond to user control of these processes. Partnership does not necessarily mean that participants have equal power, but does imply recognition and open discussion of how power is distributed and used. Some practice goes further and attempts through partnership to redistribute power between the parties, either by sharing that which is held by the more powerful or by accessing external, additional sources of power to support the less powerful. For some, only practice at this end of the partnership spectrum is worthy of the name, participation without redistribution of power being seen as an empty and frustrating process for the powerless, and as allowing policy holders to claim that all sides have been considered while only some sides benefit (Arnstein 1969). Thus, partnership must be founded on two core components: sufficient information to understand and contribute, and power to influence the outcome (Tunnard 1991). Much of what is labelled partnership practice is at best participation in worker and agency controlled agendas, and is therefore located in a two-dimensional power relationship. It clearly does have, however, the potential to engage with power issues within a three-dimensional perspective and thus contribute substantially to empowerment. This is particularly the case where users and providers join in partnership to focus attention and energy to stimulate change and movement elsewhere in an oppressive system.

Addressing barriers and defences

Subtle and pervasive processes can militate against empowerment in social care practice, the 'power of orthodoxy and convention' (Barker and Peck 1987) keeping workers and users firmly in their place. First, professional cultures are founded on the power and status of 'knowing best', speaking for others and gatekeeping access to resources, and derive role security from such actions, which do not leave room for the mechanisms of empowerment. The trappings of professional power and status are difficult to give up, particularly when the alternative is unclear, unknown and untested, appears to deny established expertise and draws on skills not yet developed. Professional insecurity and fear can manifest as defensiveness and resistance, as defeatism, over-simplification, endless debate, reliance on rhetoric and discounting of users' abilities (Braye and Preston-Shoot 1992b). Resistance also becomes institutionalized: organizational structures change only slowly to facilitate access to powerful positions, to decision-making forums (Drake 1992); top-down hierarchical bureaucracy can demonstrate a cohesion which leaves little space for negotiation or innovation, and users' voices are lost beneath mounds of policy guidance and codes of practice (Higgins 1992).

Second, users often enter the relationship with social care agencies from a structural position of powerlessness, suspicious, perhaps through previous experience, of the motives of professionals and in personal distress compounded by services which deny choice and dignity, and are sometimes underpinned by the threat of compulsion (Barber 1991). For people who have effectively long been denied the experience of exercising choice, the challenges of empowerment are greater (Ward 1991). Individuals damaged by the system purporting to help them need help to make sense of their oppression and reasons for dissent or distress (Lawson 1991). There is a strong legacy of powerlessness where power has been used to prevent people from having grievances by shaping their perceptions, cognitions and preferences, such that they accept their role in the existing order because they can see or imagine no alternative (Lukes 1974). For many users it is not merely a question of learned power positions in relation to institutionalized professional power, but of having experienced complex patterns of dominance and subordination constructed on dimensions of race, gender, class, (dis)ability, sexuality, age and health status, such that expectations and demands will be tempered by previously learned exclusion and marginalization.

The concept of internalized oppression is important here. What makes abused people accommodate to and remain with their abusers? The profound anxiety created by threats faced from the environment, such as are experienced in oppressive relationships and structures, and the impact of felt powerlessness may create resignation, acceptance of the unacceptable and a belief in the futility of action. If internalized, this may establish an attributional style characterized by personal blame ('it's all my fault'), globality ('this applies to all situations') and stability ('this will never change') (Barber 1991). Professional care workers are often puzzled when attempts to offer choice are met by users choosing more of the same, initiatives to give away power are met with dependency and offers to work in partnership elicit no dialogue.

The implications of these processes for empowerment and partnership are important. The more powerlessness is reinforced by services which deny felt experience and choice, and the more practitioners expect partnership without addressing the impact of powerlessness, the less users will be empowered. A necessary preliminary process must be engaged in, to recognize internalized oppression and address the attributional belief system which supports it. One of the major contributions of the self-advocacy movement has been to address the psychological legacy of powerlessness, to substitute different messages: 'it's not your fault', 'it does not have to be like this' and 'we can make changes'. Empowerment is far more likely when circumstances are explained by such different messages: universality ('anyone in my position would feel . . .'), transience ('this can change') and specificity ('my response is just to this situation') (Barber 1991; Rees 1991). People will only engage in partnership when they expect success, value the goals to be achieved and believe they have some control over the likelihood of realizing them.

What this analysis reveals are various barriers to empowerment: disincentives for both users and professionals (see Figure 5.4). Since the rhetoric of partnership and empowerment leaves the reality unchanged, the power to define and shape the nature and degree of participation will remain with the dominant group (Drake 1992). There are several ways in which professionals, as the dominant group, have responded to the challenge of empowerment in ways experienced as cosmetic and superficial by users and others working from a self-advocacy base. Recognizable trends include manipulation, marginalization and colonization (Beresford and Croft 1993).

Empowerment is blunted when it is viewed by professionals as merely another form of enabling (Adams 1990), when it is used on users' behalf, effectively overlooking their own power struggles (Plumb 1991). Professional colonization acts as though empowerment was solely a good professional idea, uses its mechanisms for agency purposes and denies or discounts users' part in any empowerment process. Anger at such exploitation has been expressed by black writers (REU 1990), exposing how white social care professionals draw on the knowledge and experience of black people, which is then presented as 'radical and progressive white thinking'. Even the very term empowerment does not do justice to the changes it attempts to describe. It implies the granting of a gift whereas, in reality, it is not there to be given (Gomm 1993).

Ways of manipulating mechanisms intended to enhance empowerment have been identified, particularly in relation to user involvement in planning

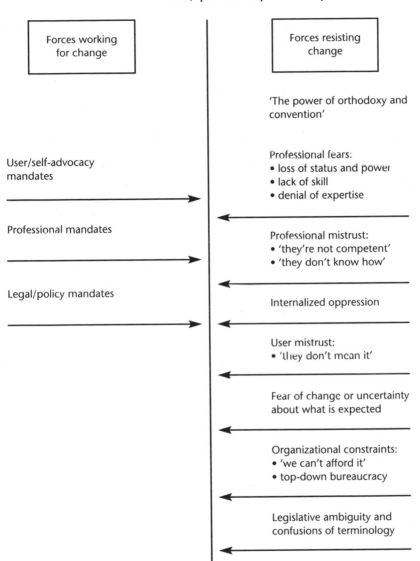

Figure 5.4 Barriers to empowerment.

and service monitoring discussions. They include (Lindow 1992; Hutchinson and McAusland 1993; User Centred Services Group 1993; Values into Action 1993b; Wallcraft 1993; Williamson 1993):

- tokenism – consultation over small aspects of issues, leaving the main decision-making with professionals;
- having user representatives on every forum of debate, with little attention to purpose or outcome;
- offering a participative place to one user, requiring that person to 'represent' others;
- challenging representativeness, indicating that users' voices are partial and therefore worth less;
- failing to divulge full and necessary information;
- keeping discussion confined to professionally set agendas, using professional jargon and protocols;
- asking for views on existing services, rather than innovation;
- not paying users for their time;
- not offering users any training in the task of planning service delivery;
- discounting users' views and feedback – 'it couldn't happen like that here';
- denying and minimizing the impact of users' experience – 'we're all disabled really' or 'we're just as powerless as you';
- setting up a users' committee by invitation, by-passing user representatives from other existing groups.

Such mechanisms produce '*managed user participation*' characterized by the following thinking:

- we're providers of services;
- we know best;
- we have to have user participation;
- let's set up a users' group;
- do you know any users we can ask?

This is a far cry from the desired alternative of '*user-managed participation*':

- get users together;
- leave us alone to talk;
- invite us to meetings;
- listen to what we say;
- give us information;
- pay our expenses (Wertheimer 1993).

Initiatives such as those described above, stemming from professional and organizational defensiveness and resistance, effectively defeat any empowering potential within them. A further set of defences is used to deny the need for such mechanisms in the first place:

- user participation takes too long, slows things down;
- we don't want to raise people's expectations;
- people don't want to be involved;
- people can use formal democratic processes for representation;

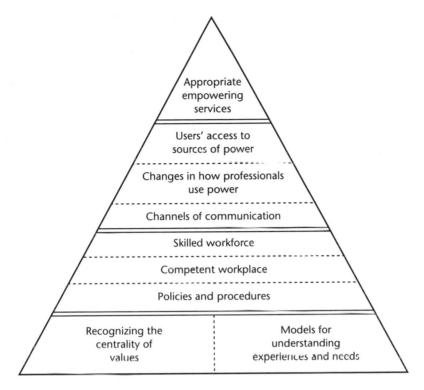

Figure 5.5 Key initiatives for empowerment.

- we don't want to burden/exploit people;
- 'they' (people in distress, people with learning disabilities, disabled people) can't do it;
- it costs too much;
- we'll do it next time;
- we do it already (Croft and Beresford 1993).

Faced with such barriers and resistance, the evolution of more empowering alternatives requires both a conducive environment and proactive initiatives for change.

Key initiatives for change

There are several important building blocks (see Figure 5.5) which combine skills, communication channels and procedures derived from a clearly articulated and understood value base, which support and sustain the gradual construction of services reflecting the principles of empowerment.

The first foundation is to recognize the *centrality of values* to practice, and the relevance of the radical value perspective in ensuring that an understanding of power and inequality in society is integrated within the value base. All practice, in effect, has a relationship with oppression. Decisions made within a dominant ideology cannot ignore their context (Dominelli 1988). It is impossible to take a neutral position. If practitioners are not part of the solution, they must be part of the problem – failing to engage with and challenge oppression condones and supports the status quo (Thompson 1993).

Developing and 'owning' a personal commitment to the values of empowerment is important for turning rhetoric into reality. This is essentially an individualized process, for practitioners will bring different mixes of socially constructed and internalized values to their work. The process of unlearning and relearning, however, is non-negotiable within the requirements for competent practice and requires active consideration of personal value assumptions in every interaction. Thus practitioners must develop an awareness of the different histories and social positions which inform their individual and collective participation in empowerment, and identify their own history of being oppressed and of participating in oppression (Husband 1991). This is necessarily a foundation for being able to work with the assumptions around which people have structured their lives, or the constructions which are placed, for example, on the experience of distress, poverty, disability or vulnerability.

Professionals are individually responsible for ensuring that good practice prevails. Lack of policy, procedure and resources should not be regarded as an excuse (B. Ahmad 1990). Empowering practice requires a personal 'will' or belief that it is possible and desirable. A powerful motivator to empowerment is the ability to stand outside one's own power position and view the potential partnership from the other's perspective. From here can be identified the fears, doubts and uncertainties which make it difficult to 'speak truth to power' (Stanton 1989), especially where race and gender dynamics add to the complexity of the interaction. It is from this position that reflection can take place upon the complexity of what is happening, the power dynamics between those involved, the relationship between the individualized distress and the wider context, between the personal and the political.

Organizations also face the challenge of asking what makes it difficult to abandon previous ways of working and to look anew at what services would meet users' needs. A further value base component in moving towards empowerment is, therefore, the commitment organizations can demonstrate to 'something different'. Central here is how organizations value their staff, since practitioners cannot empower others if they are not empowered themselves (Read and Wallcraft 1992). Since workers do not always experience this sense of empowerment, a new agency culture is required (Stevenson and Parsloe 1993), one which does more than introduce the cosmetic changes of policy statements and consultation channels, which recognizes the impact of its processes upon workers and users, and engages with them openly about how its power can be used both non-oppressively and anti-oppressively. It will submit its policies and practices to critical scrutiny, and will debate how need is defined and how services are negotiated and offered. It will be proactive in addressing areas of its service provision which have not complied with legislation such as section 71 of the RRA 1976, using these provisions to strengthen the weaker guidance in relation to appropriate community care services for black communities. Such a value commitment will be highly influential on users' experience, and can provide a counterbalance to the marginalization of less powerful groups.

Such organizational commitment has the potential to alter the power dynamic between user and agency, since it turns the spotlight on oppressive systems rather than upon the consciousness of oppressed people (Barker and Peck 1987). Ultimately, committed organizations must address the question of who defines the goals for social care, and how legislative mandates can be used with and for users rather than imposed upon them. This is not the same as saying that control is always unjust and uncaring. It points out, however, that agencies must question the norms they are asked to represent, and whether professional practice in the context of local government is compromised and asked to collude with oppression. How, for instance, an agency moves between the needs, rights, resources polarities, or the auto-nomy, protection, empowerment scenarios, will very much influence the degree of empowering practice possible. For empowerment in social care to have meaning, the organizational culture must move away from that of power (control of the expert) and role (emphasis on given tasks and pro-cedures) to that of community (learning with users). Such a culture would seek to use and enhance the power and authority held by users, while recognizing that professional power and authority remain legally mandated, and may have to be exercised.

The organizational commitment required is made more complex by the interprofessional and inter-agency agendas operating at the interface of health and social care. The policy aim of a seamless service ignores the sometimes quite different ideologies operating within agencies which may be providing simultaneous services to the same individual, and where an individualized medical response may sit uneasily with social change goals identified as part of an empowerment process. The organizational value commitment must, therefore, include the will to engage at policy level with partner agencies in discussion and negotiation about what principles will inform and drive the work.

The second foundation at this first level is the choice of *models for under-standing* users' needs and experiences. Such models are highly influential (see Chapter 2), and make a significant impact on the ethos and direction of services provided. Illness or vulnerability construed in medical terms and attributed to biological processes of ageing, disability or illness will bring an emphasis on services to 'cure' or adapt an individual's experience or response to those circumstances. Western medical models of psychiatry, or patriarchal explanations of women's distress, focused on pathology and deficiency, have created services and interventions experienced as intensely oppressive, and enabled collusion with the political role of psychiatry in containing protest and difference. Medicalizing distress and dissent obscures their origins and disempowers people (Lawson 1991). Empowering practice is founded on more holistic models which reach beyond labels of psychiatric diagnosis, physical or mental impairment and older age to gain a more personal understanding of what *this* person brings to *this* encounter; how her or his experience is constructed by her or his position within societal structures; and how social care provision can address both the personal and political dimensions of her or his experience.

If these foundations of values and models are in place, they can give rise to and support the next level, upon which are the *policies and procedures* that stem from an organizational commitment to empowerment. An effective policy framework for empowering practice will contain clear aims and objectives about both the organization's role and function and its chosen way of working with users to involve them in its operations and maximize their control. Anti-discriminatory and anti-oppressive practice principles will underpin the aims and objectives, and inform the detailed strategic steps for implementation. There will be clear monitoring criteria and procedures, geared to turning abstract rhetoric into clear, tangible results. Such policy building must tackle the challenge of turning the key aspects of the social care policy base into mechanisms for empowerment. Assessment and care management, for example, as conceptualized in government guidance, leave power and responsibility with professionals (Knapp *et al.* 1992). Agencies are responsible for redefining the professional role away from the expert rationer to a resource that users can negotiate access to (SSI 1993b), for seeing assessment as a means of providing information about what people need rather than as a means of containing demand (Ellis 1993). People's expertise on themselves and their own needs can be built into a model of assessment based on mutuality and exchange (Smale *et al.* 1993), with users as equal partners in problem definition and negotiation about solutions.

A further focus in the policy framework will be on building a *competent workplace* in which staff feel empowered. Key components will be recruitment and selection policies which reflect equal opportunity and attempt to redress the barriers to employment, training and promotion experienced by black women and men, white and black women, disabled people and others whose identifiable and visible difference makes them targets for discriminatory employment practice. Policy and procedure will be used proactively to create workplaces where racism, sexism and other forms of oppression are not tolerated, and where supportive and developmental links between groups of staff are available without question. Supervision policies will create expectations of accountability, support and learning in the workplace, and supervision and other channels will establish that the organization expects and intends to: communicate with its staff; engage in dialogue about practice; answer questions, receive feedback and incorporate that feedback into policy change and development. A policy framework in which clarity is present about aims and objectives, roles, responsibilities and channels of communication will assist individual practitioners in determining the extent and limits of their own responsibility – what individuals have control over in their practice and what is a wider issue to be addressed by the agency or to be taken up outside the agency, preferably with its support. Such understandings will also form the basis for staff development and training policies which are geared to creating a *skilled workforce*, able to overcome some of the barriers and defences identified earlier, and take on the challenge of empowerment.

A policy framework with empowerment as a central theme, and constructed on the foundation of empowering values and models, can itself be the foundation for the next tier, a major theme of which is *channels of communication*. User demands for participation have been summarized as comprising structures for access to the agency and support to use them (Beresford and Croft 1993). The communication channels must address: an individual's own use of services; mechanisms for purchasing services, ensuring money is spent on appropriate services; involvement in planning for the design and delivery of services in general; and mechanisms for monitoring quality and effectiveness (Mullender 1992/3).

Users, both as individuals and as representatives of user and community groups, have increasingly been involved in self-assessment and budget management, setting standards, recruitment and selection of staff, defining and evaluating quality, identifying and planning for required service developments and running services. Kinds of involvement vary, from that which is service- or agency-related, involving people who use a particular service such as a day centre, through participatory schemes which aim to create direct routes of communication into an agency for users or potential users, to independent user organizations which create and maintain their own membership and seek to influence statutory services through collective action (Croft and Beresford 1993). Those that are experienced as more empowering, from the perspective of promoting users' agendas, are those that are user-led rather than initiated by the organization.

Facilitation of communication is an important contribution to the effectiveness of established channels. Being able to assert views, needs and wants is a form of power, and advocacy mechanisms have a key role to play (Mind 1992), not just by being available and accessible, but also because organizations are prepared to listen and negotiate with advocates. Recognizing the limits of professional helpfulness and putting people in touch with sources of advocacy to facilitate communication is particularly important where there exists a difference of perspective and the power imbalance would otherwise allow the professional perspective to be easily imposed.

Interpreting and translating services are also essential means of facilitating communication, not through reliance on family members, children or unpaid colleagues (REU 1989), but through properly structured, trained and resourced services which are an integral part of the agency's communication systems, and are sophisticated and flexible enough to avoid the pitfalls and accommodate the subtleties of linguistic difference (Dugmore 1991). Language itself is not a neutral medium: it carries received ideas, values and standards, and is itself a form of power (Rojek *et al.* 1988). The language used as currency in channels of communication will either facilitate or stifle effective interchange of ideas and opinions. Professional and committee jargon, insistence on written communication, complex forms and documentation are all part of the professional power play which can obscure meaning and block communication.

To have even a potential chance of fulfilling objectives of empowerment, channels of communication and mechanisms for involvement must place users in a negotiating position from which power can be exercised, and where the exercise of that power has the potential to achieve its purposes (Drake 1992). An extensive literature has evolved, led by users' contributions, which detail the key characteristics and qualities required and which stress the following dimensions (Bould 1990; Winn and Chotai 1990; Read and Wallcraft 1992; Beresford and Croft 1993):

- clarity about what involvement is being offered, and what its limits are;
- involvement from the beginning in ways which are central to agency structures and processes but which are also flexible;
- tangible goals for involvement;
- involvement by choice, not compulsion;
- involvement of black and minority perspectives;
- individual and collective perspectives;
- provision of time, information, resources and training;
- openness to advocacy;
- clear channels of representation and complaint;
- involvement of key participants, not just some;
- open agendas;
- facilitation of attendance;
- emphasis on channels, particularly when rights are at risk and the agency's perspective is backed by the statutory power to impose it.

Such mechanisms have to be established proactively, and specific provision for involvement has to be made. It does not come naturally. Good intentions are not enough (Croft and Beresford 1990). An often quoted statement very effectively summarizes the value of communication channels in the process of empowerment. 'When people not used to speaking out are heard by those not used to listening, real changes can be made' (O'Brien 1989).

Two key changes form further foundations of empowerment: *changes in the way professionals negotiate and use their power* and *changes in users' access to their own sources of power*. These changes derive from and in turn enhance channels of communication. Underpinning both is the perspective of a strengths model (B. Ahmad 1990) which recognizes users' life experience and survival skills, understands experiences of oppression, works against the sources of that oppression and promotes positive images of what users bring to their encounter with professionals. Winkler (1990) notes in relation to health care that informed patients often have to renegotiate the professional–user relationship because the power they derive from knowledge upsets the traditional power balance. The same applies in social care. Power must not be obscured but viewed as a positive concept and used proactively by each party to promote his or her own and respond to the other's interests in the encounter.

A process known as principled negotiation (Isaac 1991) encapsulates this principle, and applies particularly where perspectives may differ. It focuses on interests that can be heard and deemed legitimate rather than positions that give rise to a battle of wills, and seeks to identify options which will best meet the declared interests of all parties. Such negotiations can result in the practice of using written agreements. While community care legislation (NHSCCA 1990) is silent about written agreements, policy guidance does require written records of certain procedures carried out under legislation. Assessment, for example, that results in a continuing service should be recorded as a written statement which details points of difference between the parties if agreement is not reached (DoH 1990a). Care plans should also be written (DoH 1991b) and signed by contributors to signify their agreement. Such mechanisms are important as expressions of partnership, and as a means of reflecting the principles of empowerment in everyday practice (Preston-Shoot 1994). They contribute to *establishing clarity* about the purposes of social care provision, and about the power balance between the parties to the negotiation. What level of partnership is envisaged, within which model? What is negotiable within the power relationship and what is not? What are the limits to choice, the rights and responsibilities of each party? These are vital issues to clarify in every encounter.

The *self-empowering processes* that are available to users are an important way of making a difference to how negotiation takes place, and need to be supported by recognition of two factors. One is a rejection of the idea that powerless people have to be rescued (Hearn and Morgan 1990). Channels of communication must avoid professional colonization of either the process or the content of the dialogue, and recognize that professionals cannot own, predict or regulate the results of their commitment to empowerment. The second is not to deny the obstacles that people face in taking responsibility for their own empowerment (Milroy and Hennelley 1989), whether these obstacles are through internalized oppressive experiences or structural barriers.

Collective action is a powerful counter to these factors. The processes of identifying with an oppressed group, establishing a non-individualized explanation for experiences (Shakespeare 1993) and sharing a political identity which brings the confidence to demand, not ask, for change (Bynoe *et al.* 1991) are highly effective channels of empowerment.

This analysis has identified several foundations at differing levels, all of which combine to support the provision of what might be called *appropriate services*. Appropriate here has a number of non-negotiable meanings. To be 'appropriate' in the context of empowerment, services must demonstrate the impact of the foundations identified above.

Services must be *negotiated* within the context of *overt recognition of the power relationship* between user and service provider, in a partnership that is more than just token recognition of a user's preference and within which every attempt has been made to empower the user's perspective. This will have been evident at both the overall service planning and individual provision levels.

Appropriate services will be based on a *recognition of difference*: different needs, wants, priorities and perspectives. That there is no one blueprint for services must be recognized. It is reinforced by the fact that the self-advocacy movement in mental health, for instance, argues strongly both for separatist, user-controlled services and for services run in partnership with statutory providers (Brandon 1991b). Similar differences of perspective exist within feminist practice, where concern for women-centred provision produces differing manifestations and emphases (Reynolds 1993), united by their prioritization of women's perspectives, needs and strengths, and by the centrality of gender to all the processes of decision-making underpinning provision (Hanmer and Statham 1988). Building services which recognize difference also involves addressing racial diversity and promoting developments in two dimensions. The first is the ability of statutory providers to offer services which are non-discriminatory in their availability and suitability, and are actively anti-discriminatory in tackling obstacles to equality. This means developing the ability to provide services which recognize strengths and promote positive racial and cultural identity (Jones *et al.* 1992). The second is to recognize black voluntary organizations as occupying the same role and status in relation to statutory provision as white organizations and to use funding opportunities creatively to remedy past injustices concerning the standard of service provision to black communities (Ahmad-Aziz *et al.* 1992).

Recognition of difference along the lines of social division must go alongside flexibility in being able to offer a range of provision which addresses differing needs for domiciliary, day and residential services, and is able to make varying use of combinations of services to accommodate rights to choice as well as need.

Finally, appropriate services will reflect empowerment principles in their targets of change. The focus of intervention must include change at a structural level, identifying with the cultural, social and economic experiences of a community, not just ameliorating individual distress (Milroy and Hennelley 1989). Normalization and integration work does not mean taking on the dominant values of a society. It means being able to function within that society, having a voice there, and being able to work for change without persecution (Lawson 1991). The radical change agenda needs to be balanced, though, with people's basic needs for help and support. Both structural and individual approaches are important (Adams 1990). There is a danger that the two are seen as mutually exclusive whereas, in fact, the relationship between individual need and structural agendas is intimate and complex (Braye and Varley 1992). Understanding how it operates for each individual enables need to be addressed without relying on individual pathology as a target or resource, and within the context of broader empowerment aims in relation to the individual's social network and structural position. The required balance in targets of change is summarized by Beeforth and colleagues (1990) as being one which addresses self-care, self-assertion and self-advocacy.

Within the framework suggested above, many of the traditional core skills of social care are empowering. Establishing the practice base is not a question of devising new skills, but of creating the active arenas in which conceptual understanding of empowerment can meet the belief that it is both the legitimate aim of social care and the right way to go about achieving it. It requires a reframing of the roles traditionally associated with users and professionals; the negotiation of a different relationship in which both can work together to create 'islands of empowerment in the deep and turbulent sea of social disempowerment' (Stevenson and Parsloe 1993).

Exercise 5.1. Working with Difference. When you work with someone whose gender, racial origin and/or class background is *different* from your own, what effect does this have between

you? Think of someone you are working with where differences exist, and list the effects you are aware of. Now think
what similarities and commonalities there are between you.

Now think of someone where there are broad *similarities*
in gender, racial origin or class background between you
and her or him. Now think of the differences there are –
these may be dimensions such as age, (dis)ability or social
networks, or be less obvious things like religion, sexual
preference, politics or personal history. Explore how commonality and difference in different 'divisions' can have a
differing impact on the relationship.

Exercise 5.2. Working with Difference. What have you learned, in your
family or living situation, about who has power to negotiate in what arenas – parent/child, male/female, rich/poor,
black/white, disabled/non-disabled, gay or lesbian/hetero-
sexual? How might this learning be affecting your practice?
How might you disqualify people from negotiation for partnership? How might you need to change your practice to
widen how you negotiate?

Exercise 5.3. Working in Partnership. Think of someone you are cur-
rently working with. How could you demonstrate to him or
her (over and above telling him or her verbally) that you
were keen to work in partnership? What could you do to
convince him or her? What level of partnership do you
think is possible in this situation? When you have decided,
answer the question of *why* this level, and *why not* a more
empowering level. What are the constraints or barriers? Can
you remove any of them, alone or with others?

Exercise 5.4. Partnership. Identify two people with whom you are cur-
rently working: one with whom you would say you are
working in partnership; one with whom you are not. How
did you achieve the partnership? What would you need to
change for partnership to be achieved? What can you learn
from one to apply to the other?

Exercise 5.5. Power. When in your work do you feel powerful? Where does
that power come from? How powerful are you seen by the
people you work with as service users? Where does their
perception of your power come from? When in your work
do you feel powerless? What is it like to feel that way? What
power do service users have in relation to you, your agency
and the services provided? Think of specific people if it helps.

Exercise 5.6. Power. Put yourself in the shoes of someone using your
agency's services. What would you expect from that agency

in terms of your involvement with it, its treatment of you? Now think back to your own position. How much of that expectation do you and your agency meet? What changes could be made?

Exercise 5.7.   Oppression and Empowerment. Think of a practical task you carry out in your work with a service user. List ways in which you could undertake it in an *oppressive* way. List ways in which you could do it in an *empowering* way. Are there any changes you should make to your current practice?

Part III Managing the

social care process

The chapters in this section focus upon interactive processes within social care provision. They explore those factors which enable workers to understand and manage interactions with service users, negotiate collaboratively with other professionals and agencies, and manage their personal experience of work. The emphasis is on interactions and processes, those between users and their families, between workers and users, between workers, and between agencies, which affect whether or not effective social care is achieved.

Interactions are central to social care: for example, between users and workers when gathering information, assessing need and negotiating a care package; between services when constructing and delivering a care package. Perhaps inevitably, in establishing the infrastructure for care in the community, the focus has tended to be upon key tasks. However, in devising systems for assessing needs, establishing priorities, developing the mixed economy of care, maintaining quality and delivering services, and in articulating the values which underpin social care, exactly how these tasks are to be implemented and the values expressed *in practice* has been relatively neglected. This imbalance between task and process is unfortunate. Social care involves human relationships. It requires practitioners who are committed to focusing on users' psychological well-being and relationships, and who are skilled in expressing professional values and skills alongside being competent in matching needs with resources (Davies and Missiakoulis 1988). The improvements in people's lives which effective social care can achieve, such as increased life satisfaction, greater freedom and choice, enhanced life skills and use of community facilities, require workers competent in managing such processes as engaging reluctant users, coping with challenging behaviours, blending therapeutic and basic skills, and integrating a caring attitude with a professional approach and imaginative service structures (Knapp et al. 1992; Mansell and Beasley 1993). The emphasis on key tasks and competences should not allow a mechanistic, tick-box approach to social care at the expense of creativity, imagination, intuition and reflection. It is important that practitioners retain a questioning, critical stance on how the social care task is framed and implemented if they are not to become oppressive in their interactions with users and if services are not simply to perpetuate inequalities, to reinforce existing power structures or to reproduce institutionalized forms of care.

Neither the social care task nor the process is that simple, as previous chapters will have demonstrated. The relationship between the law, values and practice is complex. The conflicting mandates and expectations held by agencies, users, carers and different professionals must be managed. Assessment and intervention will call for judgements about need versus resources, autonomy versus protection, and for the management of conflict between users and carers or between users and different agencies. There remain doubts about the potential of local and health authorities to achieve a seamless service. Nor are values always reflected in practice. Evidence exists of non-implementation of good practice statements at the interface between workers and users, even where the statements are seen as expressing what is desirable (Booth et al. 1990). In service provision, agencies continue to discriminate in terms of gender (Bebbington and Davies 1993), race and culture (Dutt 1990) and disability (Oliver 1991/2). If one lesson can be derived from the numerous reports into welfare services, it is that enquiries and subsequent legislative reforms cannot prevent tragedy. Finally, the environment in which social care practitioners and managers operate may easily be experienced as hostile. The effect of this on behaviour should not be underestimated.

Accordingly, the focus here is on managing social care, where managing means working within, coping with and negotiating the tasks and processes which are generated by community care policy, the professional value base and the practice dilemmas to which these give rise.

6 Empowering practice: understanding and managing user–worker processes

So let's take our common humanity and form a different kind of bond together where we love and respect each other where it's possible. At least not manipulate and put people down. When we do, let's be able to look at it and learn from our mistakes, learn from each other, learn new approaches. There's an incredible amount that can be done by people sitting down and listening to each other, finding out new ways of doing things – it's all there in people.

(McDonald 1992/3)

Here are two ordinary people . . . engaging in a complex transaction about 'sickness' and treatment. One is usually in pain and suffering, the other may have relevant skills and knowledge. During that transaction they contribute different perspectives and may disagree. Neither tries to manipulate the other to win control. Instead they move gently towards compromises and agreements. They move towards sharing information and respect for each other's position. They are humble rather than arrogant, aware of what they do not know rather than what they know.

(Brandon 1991b)

Achieving such relationships is not straightforward. In addition to knowledge of policy guidance and a sound value base, empowering practice in the negotiation and provision of social care requires skilled understanding of and intervention in processes which occur and influence interactions between purchasers, providers and users.

Lists abound of prerequisite values, knowledge and skills for qualifying social workers (CCETSW 1991b) and social care workers (Barclay 1982; Biggs and Weinstein 1991). They require skills in human relationships, counselling and interpersonal encounters, in assessment and analysis, in service planning and teamwork, in decision-making and rendering services accessible. Yet complications arise when people are unhappy about being assessed or receiving community care services, are unable to express their needs clearly (Huxley 1993) or are sceptical about offers of partnership. It is one thing knowing that key components of successful work include defining problems clearly, being open and honest, providing access to information and including users in decision-making; it is one thing knowing that empowerment and partnership practice requires engaging with issues of power and oppression, promoting users' skills in negotiations about the work and embracing social change goals (Braye and Preston-Shoot 1993a, b); it is quite another achieving these when people using services have experienced and continue to face disadvantage, isolation and disqualification; it is quite another when working from an agency base where statutory duties predominate and where organizational and legal structures restrict rights and participation, exercise social control and embody dominant norms (Preston-Shoot 1992).

To disentangle these complexities requires an understanding of what takes place between people. It requires an emphasis on process, recognizing that effective and equitable social care must include focusing on feelings, behaviour, relationships and psychological well-being when performing social care tasks (Davies and Knapp 1988; Bond 1992). This chapter explores the processes on which the practice of social care depends if it is to be empowering. It applies and builds upon a critical understanding of the keys to empowering practice already discussed: understanding of the policy context and the choices it offers (Chapter 1); integration of core values (Chapter 2) and the components of an enabling organizational context (Chapter 3); negotiating the complex interplay of needs, rights and resources, of autonomy, protection and welfare (Chapter 4); and the centrality of power, partnership and anti-oppressive practice (Chapter 5).

Case study

Lech Janowski is referred to a social services department by his general practitioner for services to support him with the stress of caring for his wife Maria. The couple live in a small, privately rented, unmodernized terraced house, in an urban area. The immediate locality comprises run-down private housing, a mix of older long-term residents such as the Janowskis and a more transient younger community in flats and bedsits. The community is ethnically diverse. Most people are quite poor.

The Janowskis came to Britain from Poland after the Second World War because Lech had secured employment. He had various manual jobs, and was finally made redundant in his late fifties. He is now 75. Maria is younger. Her employment history is not known. She has not been out of the house for many years and now remains in one room. Her mobility is very limited:

she moves by pulling herself from chair to bed, assisted by sticks. The doctor considers that the origin of her condition is psychosomatic, compounded now by physical inactivity. She has had one admission to psychiatric hospital, some 15 years ago, and was diagnosed as having schizophrenia.

Lech undertakes all the household tasks and Maria's personal care. He is said to be depressed and coping less and less well, with the result that the state of the house has rapidly deteriorated. He is also accumulating massive debts at local shops. He has shown the doctor bruises where his wife hits him if he has been too long away from the house. The doctor believes that Lech is deeply unhappy and is considering leaving his wife.

The Janowskis have no children and are said to be very isolated within their local community as a result of their reclusive existence. Lech's English is limited: he understands more than he speaks. Maria does not speak at all. It is unclear whether she understands English. All communication with her is through Lech, and is mainly non-verbal.

Exercise 6.1.   Think about the information outlined above. What are the tasks facing social care professionals? What legislation and policy guidance is relevant here? How might a value base of empowerment inform what is done in this situation?

Local authorities have a duty to assess need and to decide whether this calls for the provision of community care services (section 47, NHSCCA 1990). The doctor's concern means that their eligibility for assessment is unlikely to be doubted. More uncertain, however, is the required level of assessment. The local authority's own guidelines and procedures will be crucial in determining the scale and nature of assessment, and who undertakes it. At one level, the doctor's request may be interpreted as a need for domiciliary services, with a focus on practical provision that would provide respite for Lech in his caring role. At a covert level, an agenda may well be present to 'patch up' a vulnerable caring situation which, if it breaks down, could give rise to rapidly escalating and costly services. Alternatively, at the other extreme, a need may exist for a more substantial assessment, which might encompass physical, emotional and environmental needs, and an assessment of mental health, perhaps resulting in a range of differing resources. The wider the assessment focus, the more complex it will become, and an agency keen to empower service users will guard against limiting eligibility for full assessment as a means of rationing services.

Policy guidance clearly requires assessment to be multidisciplinary, and to involve users and carers. Who is the user in this situation? Can Lech and Maria be seen as a 'couple' with needs in common? If not, whose needs should be prioritized? Should provision designed to meet the needs of one be negotiated with the other? There is clearly scope here, as in many situations, to make things worse for one person while ameliorating the position of another. The multidisciplinary network is also, potentially, complex. There are hints in the information given that a range of differing perspectives may be valuable here. Have health care needs been fully investigated? Does the diagnosis 'psychosomatic' mean an end to enquiries as to physical health? How might mental health be assessed? What wider social and environmental needs might exist? It is not the purpose of this discussion to explore the content of the assessment in detail. The concern here is more with the values that inform what is thought, said and done.

Power

Exercise 6.2.   What are the patterns of power in the situation described? Who has what power and why? What are the potential uses and abuses of these power positions?

The relationship between Lech and Maria indicates several possible power dynamics between them: Lech as a white man, with the status of 'husband', economic power within the relationship, his links outside the home, his communication ability; Maria as a woman attempting to exercise some control or protest through physical violence in the context of her apparent dependency. The complexity of the power dynamic between them will be fed by the history of their relationship and feelings, upon which initial assessment is unlikely to touch, yet which are integral to why things are as they are. Consider also the degree of accommodation that has gone on, the one to the other, in the context of their perceived power position in relation to the other, and the degree to which they may have internalized oppression experienced from or associated with the other.

Widening the power analysis, this relationship exists in a patriarchal society where images and stereotypes of gender relations influence how they are seen by others, and for the Janowskis themselves are superimposed upon expectations and values from their culture of origin. Consider too Lech and Maria's position in their community. Do they have a community? What is their status: 'former Polish immigrants' or 'local citizens'? Are they connected to channels of identity, support and assistance? What is the status of the community in which they live in relation to wider society?

What, moreover, of the power relations *vis-à-vis* professional involvement with the Janowskis? From the information given it appears that they have seldom benefited from professional attention. Why is this? Has there been discrimination in service provision? Professionals previously involved may have known little about their background, needs, wants or aspirations. How has communication taken place, with whom, in what language? Professionals have had the power to define Maria as having schizophrenia and a psychosomatic illness. Upon what knowledge has this been based? What assumptions might have been made based on culturally normative expectations or stereotypical responses to women's mental health?

In the context of the ethos of consumerism in community care services, how far have the Janowskis been consulted so far about either how they view their own situation or what call they may wish to make on services? Do they know of this referral? Is the doctor's agenda their agenda? Would they have felt safe to disagree? Social care workers who may become involved at this point have similar power potential: status as professionals, skills and knowledge, the power to define and to gatekeep resources, to work in partnership or as 'experts', to involve the Janowskis in collaboration or to impose solutions. Workers themselves will be of specific racial and ethnic origin, male or female, of varying socio-economic backgrounds – factors bringing dimensions of similarity and difference between them, both within the professional network and in relation to the Janowskis, which in themselves will influence the power dynamics at work.

Power and influence are easy to overuse or abuse by dint of workers' positional status and legal mandates, knowledge, user demands, or a personal investment – the helping profession syndrome (Preston-Shoot and Agass 1990), where a worker's unmet needs are assuaged by compulsive care-giving. This can reinforce passivity, resistance, defensiveness, dependence and hierarchy. Indeed, users sometimes complain of professional bossiness (Booth *et al.* 1990), a disempowering assumption of responsibility, control and decision-making. It fails to allow people to see their own experiences or to reach their own conclusions on how to tackle these effectively. Central to empowering practice are questions about power in each situation, not making automatic assumptions about where power lies, about who is or is not powerful.

Images

Exercise 6.3.   Review the information given about Lech and Maria. What are the value assumptions that could be made about them, individually and together? What are the dominant images available about 'people like them'?

Since the 1960s in particular Britain has developed very hostile immigration policies. Many of the more punitive and restrictive measures have been reserved for black people, but Lech and Maria may not have escaped hostility, particularly in times of economic restraint and high unemployment, housing shortage and health care retraction. Both the assimilationist expectation that people who are 'different' will adapt and blend in with the majority, and the pluralist respect for cultural diversity, are challenged by the Janowskis, who have neither lost nor celebrated their Polish origins, and are members of neither community. Additionally, they are poor, they owe people money and their house and clothes are dirty. What images does this conjure up? What are the stereotypes that could influence how they are viewed?

Alternatively, what images abound in relation to a man in Lech's position: he fought for the Allies in the war, worked hard all his life, has devoted himself to his wife's care, is abused by her for his pains. Are there tempting stereotypes here? Would they be the same if the positions were reversed and the hardworking wife was caring for a demanding husband? Moreover, what of Maria? Why is so much less known about her? Is she seen as a person in her own right or as an appendage, a drain on her husband and potentially the state?

Images of mental health and illness potentially affect both Maria and Lech. What might be expected of someone who has been in psychiatric hospital, someone who is depressed, someone who has a psychosomatic illness? There may well be temptations to assume less competency, less understanding, more risk, more trouble, less partnership, in the presence of such factors.

Models

Exercise 6.4.   What are the different possibilities for understanding what is happening in this situation, the different explanations for why things are as they are? What models for understanding underpin those explanations?

Medical, psychosocial and social/structural models may all have relevance here, and might certainly inform the perspectives of differing professionals involved. At a simplistic level, medical explanations could be brought to bear on both Lech and Maria's mental health, searching for the biological origins, and perhaps offering pharmocological treatment, for both Lech's 'depression' and Maria's 'schizophrenia'. Psychosocial perspectives are often superimposed, emphasizing the role of stress factors in triggering a condition for which there is already some biological predisposition. Characteristic of such explanations is their linear nature, as if cause and effect can be established along the lines of human equation building.

Explanations of Maria's physical impairment may contain similar factors, either a search for a medically identifiable physical cause or, in its absence, psychological explanations which draw similarly on individual pathology and linear causality.

Social and structural models will widen the frame considerably. Lech's 'depression' may be seen as a response to the powerlessness he may experience, in relation to both his domestic role and his social and economic position in the community. Attempts to apply such a perspective to Maria's position will require a whole range of questions to be considered. What was her experience of coming to Britain originally? What did she leave behind? What expectations did she have, both in her relationship with Lech and of her life here? How far have these been met? Might her 'condition' be seen as a protest against hostility and discrimination from the community, or as a response to interactions within her relationship with Lech? Are the labels that have been attached the result of assumptions and misunderstandings made by those with the power to define, or attempts to contain and treat troublesome, threatening, ill-understood and tolerated expressions of legitimate and understandable distress?

Right answers might not exist, nor simple ways of understanding what is happening in this situation. However, it is important to retain an open mind, an awareness that the obvious explanation may not be the only one, that alternatives exist and may prove fruitful in creating options for the focus of any approach and intervention.

Preparation for approaching the Janowskis

Exercise 6.5.   Imagine yourself to be Lech or Maria in the context of this referral. How might you be feeling? What anxieties and questions might you have? What might you be worried about? What would you want to know? How would you want professionals to behave towards you?

The ability to shift perspective, to stand in the shoes of people needing social care services, to appreciate how they might experience this encounter, is an important part of preparing to approach people who use, or may wish to use, services. It is important to identify the potential concerns Lech and Maria may have, and to recognize those they may share and those they may hold alone, perhaps hidden from the other. Do we want or welcome this attention? Who is coming to see us? Will we understand them, will they understand us? What will we have to do and say? How much will we have to tell them? Will they want to listen? How well will they explain things? Will I have a chance to talk to them on my own? Will I have to see them alone?

Doing this exercise may evoke feelings of anger, uncertainty, reluctance, fear, relief, a wish to be heard and validated as well as to keep some things private, all of which may mirror what is experienced by people using services, and which give rise to reactions sometimes experienced by practitioners as hostile, resistant, unreasonable or demanding. How initial approaches are made and the interactions managed is therefore crucial to establishing a framework which can be positive and constructive.

Exercise 6.6.   Imagine you are meeting the Janowskis for the first time, perhaps as a worker responsible for facilitating an assessment of need and a care package, or perhaps as a practitioner responsible for providing domiciliary services as part of a care package. What factors would be important to how you approach your initial encounters with them?

Establishing a working relationship requires preparation, time and skill. Images or past experiences of welfare professionals, including the loss of significant working relationships, or feelings of guilt and shame, may discourage initial or ongoing involvement. Alternatively, users may feel overwhelmed or out of control of their situation, which may result in professionals being flooded with information and demands for action. Users may anticipate, bring to or impose on this encounter previous experiences of relationships with care-givers. Where these have been characterized by unresponsiveness, anxiety, violence or an absence of security and reliability, the defences used to cope then may resurface in new relationships, whatever their quality, in declining assistance, lack of trust and failed appointments. If workers are not to see these patterns as resistance, hostility and low motivation, and to act out feelings and roles associated with such responses, what is happening must be understood and reflected back.

Even without the complications of previous experience, reservations about engaging are natural. Lech and Maria may be anxious about how they will be perceived, whether they will be liked and whether they are safe to discuss problems. This may be expressed through ambivalence in engaging in a relationship, testing a worker's understanding and reliability while preserving some part of oneself from involvement. These feelings should be addressed – finding out about how the Janowskis perceive the encounter and their previous involvement with health and welfare professionals, enquiring directly and offering experience of what can happen around opening encounters.

Preparation also requires agreeing the basis for working together. Where compulsion features in the referral, for instance statutory duties, this should be discussed openly. Room for manoeuvre will doubtless be limited but the choices, and their implications, should be explored. Even where compulsion does not underpin involvement, there may none the less be an important distinction between what is or is not negotiable, and the powers and duties workers have and the circumstances in which they may be invoked. The inability to guarantee absolute confidentiality of information is one illustration; another is the restrictions on users' rights of access to information held about them. Equally, to minimize defensiveness and ambiguity in the relationship, workers should 'set the scene' – clarify why contact is occurring, the principles by which they work, how partnership is practised. They should present reasons and/or evidence for the effectiveness of what they propose, and negotiate such matters as time, venue, frequency and purpose of contact.

The referrer's position and the referral's timing may provide useful information about a situation. Some referrals present one person as the problem, say Maria, when closer enquiry may uncover that this is to avoid conflict between other people, say Lech and the doctor. Some referrals are vague or provide minimal information. In others referrers unambiguously present the solution required and invite assent, but closer consideration of the context might indicate that others will have different views about relationships and options for change. Maria may not agree with Lech and the doctor's preferred solution. Focusing on the interactions between referrer and referred, and/or within the wider network, is essential to avoid inappropriate alliances with one party and his or her focus, and by implication criticism of the other party. Professional systems can share the same characteristics, with referrals possibly masking disagreement between agencies or defensive practice. Key questions are useful here. What is the problem and its possible meaning or function? Why has the referral been made now? Who referred and why? What different ways are there of considering the presenting problem? Different people may have different perceptions of the problems and/or change required. Such differences should be explored, using positive reframing

whereby a different perspective is given to what people are defining negatively, or frees people from previously held perspectives, as a basis for negotiating goals and changes acceptable to those involved. Positive reframing
allows change to occur without people having to accept error or blame.

Relationship building will draw extensively on traditional values of respect
and empathy, while incorporating both an anti-discriminatory and an anti-
oppressive perspective. Careful consideration of issues such as the gender of
the worker, the language in which discussions take place and the offer of
joint or single discussions will contribute to setting a framework for service
provision that does not discriminate. Recognizing areas of similarity and
difference between the individuals involved and working both to establish
commonality and to respect and deal with difference will be important, and
potentially challenging to workers as closer involvement may reveal differences between Lech and Maria themselves.

An important factor in building relationships that can take the work forward will be the degree to which workers can recognize not just the needs
or deficits in Lech and Maria's situation but also the strengths, the coping
and survival that have brought them this far, and the ways in which these
can be turned to resources in the current situation.

An approach based on partnership implies care being taken not to enter
the situation with preconceived notions of what is 'the truth' about what is
happening, and to remain as open as possible to exploration of diverse
agendas from both professionals' and users' perspectives. The approach is
perhaps best described as one of 'concerned curiosity' (Cecchin 1987) which
explores all possibilities, delaying action until varying perspectives are fully
understood, even when pressure is applied for more immediate action.

With users as experts on the content of their situation, and with users and
workers both bringing problem-solving expertise, one task for workers is to
negotiate the level of their involvement: when to be central and when peri-
pheral. They must be clear when and why responsibility must be assumed,
when a needs-led service involves non-negotiable legal duties and professional-led decisions to intervene. Otherwise, confusion will exist about the
level of partnership which is mandated and can be developed.

A non-exploitative relationship with the Janowskis will be characterized by
workers having identified the dual nature of their accountability: communicating the agency's roles and tasks to Lech and Maria, and their views to
the agencies involved. They will have discussed their authority, the extent
of the mandates they carry and the principles governing their use, together
with what authority Lech and Maria perceive them to have in their situation
and any anxieties they may have about their involvement. They will have
shared areas of concern, where possible prioritizing Lech and Maria's aims
for work, acting on their problem definition and analysis rather than press-
ing for particular decisions.

One key feature of empowering practice will be agreement based on the
phase of the work and level of trust established. Given that trust may require
time to develop, as may clarity about the work's purposes and the resources
(agency, worker, user) available, agreements may require revision and development, indicating initially the areas for further discussion and elaboration

alongside those where assessment has been completed and decisions have been made (Corden and Preston-Shoot 1987). Agreements must be negotiated with particular safeguards: confronting any pressure users may feel to comply with worker interpretations or suggestions; 'cooling-off' periods where the parties may reconsider what has been negotiated; and advocacy.

Agreeing the basis of work requires listening and demonstrating concern and capacity to understand people's experiences (Smale *et al.* 1993). People are equal partners in negotiating how problems and solutions are defined – a partnership approach markedly different from assessment to ascertain if users' needs match set criteria, or from workers producing questions and solutions without explanation. The objective is to achieve the following key ingredients for effective work:

- Clearly defined problems with specific objectives and tasks precise enough to provide a clear and agreed focus expressed in a formulated agreement.
- Openness and honesty, with differences of opinion and power imbalances addressed openly, and the work's purposes clearly understood.
- Active support of significant people in the worker–user environment.
- User involvement in problem definition, decision-making and reviews to ensure the work's continuing clarity and relevance, and to acknowledge that users are the best assessors of their own needs. Decisions should be made on hard information and negotiation, to preserve independence where possible and to reduce risks (Rogers 1990).
- Clarity on the extent to which there is full agreement on the issues to be tackled and the means by which this will be done, or whether the goals may differ but there is sufficient common ground for people to feel able to commit themselves to working towards each other's aims (Corden and Preston-Shoot 1987).
- Identifying and using users' own resources, strengths and skills for objectives to which they feel able to commit themselves.
- Clarity about the target of intervention. The focus of work may not be the individual but wider systems of which the individual is a part (family) or which impact on her or him (community attitudes, agency policies) (Barber 1991). The focus of work with these wider systems may be informed by issues presented by one individual and/or by themes arising from work across several social care situations. Both involve developing community networks and resources, such as day care, leisure services, education opportunities and employment (Knapp *et al.* 1992), so that these may be linked to individual needs as appropriate. This helps to promote integration, belonging and relationships, important elements when the fragmentation of relationships (Hatfield *et al.* 1992/3), isolation and negative aspects of community life and attitudes (Payne 1987) can undermine choice, autonomy and esteem.

Maria's story

You must not think that what you see is the truth. Everyone thinks he is wonderful to look after me as he does. You do not hear him shout and torment me when he has been out drinking. You do not feel his hands on you as I do, hurting me for his pleasure. And you wonder that I hit out when I can? He has kept me a prisoner here, broken my spirit until I have lost the will and the hope that things can be different. I came with such high hopes – work, a home, children. We lost everything back home – what do you know of my life in Poland? How can you imagine what we went through? Yet even now I long to return. My whole body hurts now, I cannot move even if I wanted to. There is no point.

Lech's story

I do my best to look after her, but you can have no idea how difficult she is. She will shout and scream at me to do things for her, then not speak for days on end. She infuriates me because she will speak to no one else, she has never bothered to learn English, kept herself to herself all these years, expects me to do everything. I know she could walk if she wanted to. I am sad for her, though, and for us, for our life together here. She is all I have left and I all she has – she would allow no one else to care for her. I must keep going as long as I can. I think the doctor has not understood me – I could never leave her, however much she hurts me. I just wish she would understand I need to get out for a drink sometimes. She thinks I see other women – it's part of her illness. She so wanted children but it never happened and she blames herself.

Self-awareness

Exercise 6.7.   If you were working with Lech and Maria, with whom would you most identify? For what reason? What elements of this situation might generate strong feelings in you, and why?

Preparation for and review of practice requires workers to understand themselves, their relationship with and impact on others, and their strengths and weaknesses in relation to maintaining a professional role. In the Janowskis' case this includes the ability to recognize their bias and feelings, how they may determine or limit the options perceived for intervention. Such responses, if left unexamined, will leave practitioners unable to identify or challenge assumptions around which others have structured their lives or the constructions those with power place on such matters as family life, gender, caring, mental distress and race (Preston-Shoot and Agass 1990). Personal bias and experience may also influence professional responses to alleged abuse and violence, such as that raised by both Maria and Lech's doctor.

Practice is affected by more than personal values and attitudes. The complexity of human interaction can trigger personal responses and associations – memories and unresolved feelings, perhaps long-hidden. These can block effective work. Situations encountered at work may resemble a worker's own family situation. Work may involve powerful emotions – aggression, hostility, sadness, pain – such that retaining a professional role becomes stressful and difficult. Taking and communicating difficult decisions cannot be avoided and yet will evoke anxiety and stress, against which workers may defend by: minimizing their authority or being authoritarian and emphasizing conformity to guidelines and procedures; prescribing solutions based on preconceptions before understanding the problems being presented; avoiding expression of emotions (Preston-Shoot and Agass 1990). The concept of professional dangerousness (DoH 1988) encapsulates these phenomena: colluding to avoid particular issues or situations; becoming over-involved or over-identified with all or some of the people involved; not recognizing or dealing with personal feelings or reactions. Workers here are unresponsive, self-preoccupied, acting ineffectively with their environment. If they are to avoid withdrawing, feeling overwhelmed or defeated, or to avoid defensiveness and acting out their reactions inappropriately, creating perhaps escalating hostility between themselves and users, if they are to remain open, responsive and effective, they too must feel empowered.

These processes may be understood as two forms of counter-transference: personal and diagnostic (Casement 1985). Both provide information about the worker's side of the interaction. Personal counter-transference refers to the worker's own reactions determined by her or his own personal history and current experience. These reactions can distort understanding of what is happening or needed. Diagnostic counter-transference refers to reactions and roles aroused in workers by users' projections, when workers are cast in particular roles which, if left unaware, are taken on. The task in both cases is to understand the process as communication of information about oneself and/or the user's world, and to avoid acting out any role projected by the user. This requires self-examination and supervision, to arrive at an understanding of what is going on within the worker, and between worker and user.

One useful approach is to develop an internal supervisor (Casement 1985), standing back or stepping outside oneself to monitor work and the complex processes or dynamics entailed within it. This may help workers to avoid becoming part of the problem. The following questions need to be asked.

- What is happening?
- What part am I playing or expected to play?
- What do I feel about this?
- What am I most anxious about in terms of my role, tasks, others involved?
- What might they be anxious about in terms of my role, tasks, their role?
- What do I find difficult in these situations and why?
- What helps me to cope?
- Are there key experiences which shed light on my difficulties in these situations and make it difficult for me to respond professionally?

Another useful strategy is to complete a personal profile and resources questionnaire (Preston-Shoot 1987). The questions may be both general and specific to particular methods or areas of work. Thus:

- What would you or your colleagues say are encouraging patterns in how you work?
- What resources (values, knowledge, skills, experiences) do you bring to the work?
- What would you say are your strengths and learning needs?
- What skills are you confident in and what areas do you want to develop?
- What are your feelings about . . .?
- What experiences have you had in . . .?

Dealing with difficult situations may prove somewhat easier if workers are confident in their own resources, and accompany this with preparation about what they want from and might encounter in particular interactions.

A third element is to review personal learning and development, personal strengths and resources, and training needs. Not knowing or experiencing doubt, uncertainty and confusion can all be positive features of learning. Without a capacity or opportunity to reflect, chaos or 'stuckness' may follow.

Managing ongoing processes

Resistance

Resistance is a pejorative term, carrying negative connotations in which it is easy to become embroiled, evidenced by anger towards the user. What the worker experiences as resistance may be reframed as service users exercising autonomy and choice about their involvement with service providers. The problem is that by assessment sufficient concern may have been aroused to lead professionals to the possibility of not withdrawing from the situation. Stepping back and putting oneself in their shoes, and considering what is being communicated on the basis of that perception, might provide useful information. Resistance may be connected with purposes and goals: objectives and solutions might feel too large, unattainable and requiring further division, or there may no longer be agreement about them. The goals may not be perceived as relevant or valuable, or the methods to achieve them might be unclear or unacceptable. It may reflect ambivalence about the change process. Even with safeguards built into agreements and care plans, allowing revision, it will be difficult for users to know what to expect. They may remain unsure what the proposed intervention will involve. Change can be experienced as painful. Whatever has precipitated contact with welfare agencies will have evoked feelings, and may raise anxieties about whether the change now sought will result in 'calamities' which previously acted as restraints on change. These fears, when present, may need to be acknowledged and worked through.

Moving from the individual to a focus on the individual in context, the resistance may come from the 'loser in the system', perhaps from one party who perceives his or her individual needs and wants being ignored. Here again, these possibilities should be reflected back, acknowledging conflicting interests, strained relationships and difficult choices about freedom and risk. This effective challenging (Smale *et al.* 1993) may raise the worker's anxieties since confronting power in a system or raising difficult issues can prove stressful. This connects back to self-awareness and to positive reframing, as strategies for personal survival and effective working. Workers may also find circular questioning (Stratton *et al.* 1990) useful here: asking involuntary users 'what needs to happen, what can you do, to help other people not to be so concerned about you?'

Closeness and distance

Professional intervention can be disabling. Knapp and colleagues (1992) chronicle what people with learning disabilities being considered for resettlement in the community could not do in terms of communication, personal care, living skills, behaviour and emotional well-being. Clearly, effective social care requires relationships and services which provide stimulation and meet social needs as well as offer basic care (Challis *et al.* 1988). For example, using day care groups in a carer's home, based around meals, can break down isolation and overcome diet neglect. Survival in the community is associated with the existence of structured plans for care and after-care (Schneider 1993) and access to imaginative services. However, two balances must be struck here.

First, workers will have to engage with feelings associated with providing physical care, with painful aspects of work, and handle the emotional content generated in themselves or within users. Emotions are not inappropriate and cannot be avoided in caring relationships. However, if control of emotions is not to result in undue distance or rejection, workers themselves must feel 'held'. The feelings (held by workers and users) and dynamics associated with physical care, often of an intimate nature, should be discussed openly in supervision, with additional debriefing after distressing or critical incidents. If the emotional content of caring is not to become over-burdening, because of its proximity, physical content, dependency, unpredictability or unnerving predictability, such regular reviews are necessary, discussing how to ensure that the experience of receiving social care is empowering and personalized, and that the experience of providing social care does not result in over-protectiveness or discouragement of necessary dependence because of the worker's anxieties. The former involves distinguishing between negotiation and what might justify protection, and between those aspects of daily living that have emotional significance for themselves and users and those that do not (Stevenson and Parsloe 1993). The latter focus involves consideration of motives, pressures and anxieties influencing what workers want to achieve.

The second balance relates to the worker–user relationship. Workers can over-care, or confuse detrimental with constructive dependency (Purtilo 1993). If over-identified, the worker cannot see the other person as an individual but only through stereotypes or counter-transference reactions. If entangled, the worker is more likely to engage in mindless doing than to act thinkingly. Dagnan and Drewett's finding (1988) that people with learning disabilities in family care homes were less likely to learn community-oriented living skills is just one example of the importance of prioritizing gains in independence, drawing realistic boundaries and expectations.

Holding

Workers must sometimes act as containers for the feelings associated with dependence, for the hurt feelings, since change lies in helping users to recognize and express uncertainty, conflict, pain, emptiness and the defences used to mask these. Accordingly, care managers and purchasers must be travel companions rather than travel agents (Renshaw 1988; Onyett 1992), having sufficient contact and rapport to manage both the task and relationship issues. Establishing and maintaining collaborative partnerships requires commitment to relationships. Providers too must work to create a stable and continuous relationship, creating a context where development and change can occur. Creating confiding relationships (Davies 1988) does have a powerful effect on morale; matching services to needs is insufficient to promote independent living or reduce unnecessary admissions to residential care. Purchasers and providers cannot eliminate all anxiety, pain, uncertainty and distress but they can create an underlying security (Kitwood and Bredin 1992) that needs will be held and met at a physical and emotional level through a structured plan with clear objectives. This provides confidence for users to express emotions, initiate contact and enjoy acceptance. Thus, containing anxiety, anger, sadness and grief is an important skill, with the aim of opening up the process of understanding and discussion where feelings can be reintegrated in a more manageable form. When responded to in this way, feelings appear more manageable; otherwise anxiety, and responses to it, may become out of control.

Advocacy

Workers will sometimes act directly as advocates, either to help people use their power, or to articulate other's needs as they perceive them, to secure the services they require and/or the rights to which they and their advocate believe them to be entitled, such as to support and information, or the normality of risk and independence, or to a positive but safe attitude to risk-taking (Williamson 1993). Advocacy is designed to redress power imbalances, say between purchasers and users, by facilitating discussion of options, dissent and review of the content of negotiated agreements.

Various approaches to advocacy exist. One distinction is between issue and case advocacy, where the former may involve groups of users; another is between lay advocacy, using skilled volunteers supported by an independent agency, paid advocacy, using skilled workers supported by an independent agency, and self-advocacy, users separately or collectively advocating on their own behalf (Barker and Peck 1987). This second set of distinctions implicitly recognizes the limitations of professional helpfulness owing to workers' location within agencies. Agencies and their employees must recognize the inevitable restrictions on the advice and support through negotiations which they can provide when they themselves are the 'other party' to the negotiations. Consequently, a key to empowering practice is connecting people to other sources of support and advocacy, while providing information about the people to engage with in the organization in order to gain access to agency decision-making processes. None the less, many users will have limited experience of dealing with bureaucracies (Knapp *et al.* 1992). If practitioners develop good working relationships with these systems, and maintain their communication and negotiation skills, they will be better placed to advocate for resources for users. Equally, they may use their groupwork skills to bring together advocacy groups, such as residents' groups, to enable users to comment on services received. Groups provide an important source of collective strength, although, once again, workers must be careful to negotiate their role with users.

Consent

Implicit throughout this discussion is the notion of consent. Too often it is assumed, and people are encouraged to communicate when they are not giving it (O'Sullivan 1990), a step which some may feel is too unsafe to take. Except where non-negotiable duties to intervene exist, people should be asked for their active consent to intervention. In some circumstances workers may feel that neither consent nor agreements can be made validly. However, both are possible (Corden and Preston-Shoot 1987; Fisher 1990b). Where passive consent is used, records must indicate the communication methods used and their outcome. Workers should continue to seek consent, watch for resistance which may indicate its absence and ensure that services provided are relevant to users' needs. Passive consent may be combined with a 'substitute judgement' test, whereby professionals act on an understanding of what someone might have wanted to happen had she or he been able to make active agreements. This is not unproblematic. Who decides? What if the decision is harmful? What if the individual has been abused or coerced by others? These problems are not insurmountable. Memory aids, reminiscence, interpreting small signs and the careful collation of historical information might yield valuable insights into the person. Practice should incorporate: honesty, avoiding deception, coercion and duress; non-confrontation, respecting and seeking to understand a person's reality; involvement, not excluding people from the knowledge that a decision is necessary or from information, given verbally and non-verbally, to make informed decisions by helping them to process reality, to understand and react realistically to it (Payne 1987). Independence and acceptable risks should be encouraged, recognizing (Rogers 1990) that this involves a balance, since obviating some risks, such as hazards at home, raises others, like prognosis on admission to residential care. The balance may be better struck when assessment focuses on utilizing an individual's strengths and when protective intervention on the grounds of an individual's incapacity is as limited as possible (Law Commission 1993).

Identifying distress

A likely challenge to service providers, especially those in positions where frequency and depth of contact creates a relationship of some intimacy and trust, will be to respond to expressions of distress and, sometimes, despair. Mental health problems are often assumed to be the province of specialist services, requiring special knowledge and skills within the realms of psychiatry. While this may be true of acute situations involving major deviations from everyday behaviour and reality, more commonly the opportunity to respond to anxiety, depression and other manifestations of distress is more likely to be presented to social care workers. Theirs may indeed be the response which makes a difference to the sense of fear and isolation commonly described by people in distress, irrespective of whether there is additional involvement with formal psychiatric services.

A mental health perspective is thus important in social care practice. This includes: recognition of the distress that individuals experience and of the need for a response to that experience on a personal level; recognition of the social and structural factors in society which impact upon and define an individual's experience, and of the need for a response at an environmental level; and recognition of how mental health services can themselves be put to oppressive purposes (Braye and Varley 1992).

At an initial response level, people in distress have the same needs as anyone else for contact, understanding, acceptance and respect. The use of non-verbal contact, empathetic statements and enquiries about feelings and thoughts, picking up on verbal clues and following what has been said rather than sticking to a preset discussion agenda, asking open but focused questions: these are all behaviours which enhance the likelihood of identifying someone's distress (Goldberg and Huxley 1992). The impact of adverse life events on mental health and levels of distress is well established, but social care workers are particularly well placed to identify the vulnerability factors in people's lives which can increase the rate and the impact of such events, and to enhance and mobilize protective factors.

It is also likely that social care workers will encounter situations of heightened distress, such that self-harm or suicide are possibilities that must be considered. Reducing suicide is a key Department of Health target, and training people working in frontline contact with vulnerable people is a priority. Certain factors might alert one to the possibility of suicide: loss, bereavement, abuse, serious illness, accompanied perhaps by changes in thinking, feeling or behaviour. Sometimes there is a self-harm content to conversation, or apparent preparation for suicide by putting things in order. Engaging trust, through reliability and acceptance, and identifying risks are key factors, openly addressing the question of whether suicide is contemplated. Workers often feel they should hang back from asking, whereas in reality there is nothing to lose and everything to gain. Key indicators of high risk are: a plan, particularly if preparations have been made and the means are available; prior suicidal behaviour or a family history of such; and low resources, isolation or lack of support.

Often a frontline worker's response will be the crucial factor which makes the 'just noticeable difference' (Schneidman 1985) to the potentially lethal mix of heightened distress and intention to die. The key to making this difference is helping the person gain a degree of control over processes which are out of control:

- attempting to reduce the impact of whatever is causing such emotional pain;
- finding a way in the short term to meet frustrated needs;
- helping to find alternative solutions, other ways of achieving what is sought through death;
- offering the prospect of hope;
- removing the means;
- involving others to support;
- recalling previous successful coping mechanisms;
- playing for time – 'not today';
- making yourself important to the person and asking for a commitment;
- setting small specific objectives and tasks.

Supporting people through emotional crisis makes considerable demands on a worker's resources, and entails needs for support, both during and after the process. This can mean a range of things, from extra time with the service user to time and space for the worker to share the impact of the work. These resources will be discussed in Chapter 8.

Recording

One feature of partnership is open records. Access to records is endorsed in law (see Chapter 4) but shared recording is not. However, involving users in recording is a mark of empowering practice and reflects the need for a redefinition of ownership of information (Beeforth *et al.* 1990). Workers are often pressurized into recording in ways which do not render local authorities liable to provide services. Equally, records are too often constructed haphazardly, failing to use available information to form a coherent and comprehensive picture, with assessment indistinguishable from running records (SSI 1993b). Recording is an important tool for working in partnership and for informing practice. It should clarify how questions of rights, risks and choice have been decided, how the assessment was undertaken and how the care plan relates to the information obtained. Records, jointly constructed, should identify relevant historical information and use this alongside new information to identify themes, patterns and needs. One record is preferable, with all professionals pooling their knowledge to avoid the pitfalls of missing relevant information. User involvement and empowerment will be facilitated further if the user holds the record (Fisher 1990b).

Leaving

It should not be assumed that, once assessed as necessary, social care services will continue to be provided. Situations change. Emphasizing services to promote people's strengths, and ensuring that planning and action are directed towards purposeful outcomes, valued by users and carers, implies regular review of provision. Where reviews conclude by agreeing withdrawal of services, this should be achieved gradually, to allow the parties to disengage from relationships and to consolidate achieved change. Focusing on content, on completion of tasks, should not neglect the possibility of feelings that work is terminating because of some fault on the user's part.

Where work continues but the workers change, this must be handled sensitively. Strong, trusting relationships, built with one worker, are not easily relinquished or transferred to another. The loss of significant relationships can result in previous difficulties or issues reappearing, in reactivation of strong feelings about previous relationships or in the presentation of new problems. The emotional impact of change, the uniqueness and meaning of the situation for *this* individual, should be centre stage.

Workers too may experience difficulty relinquishing relationships, irrespective of whether the change is voluntary or the result of agency policy. There should be opportunities, through supervision and staff care, for workers to share the impact of change, with particular reference to leaving ongoing situations.

7 Understanding and managing the interprofessional system

Empowering social care practitioners and users must include using frameworks to understand and secure interprofessional and inter-agency collaboration. People working together require systems for communication, collaboration and decision-making, yet negotiating, establishing and maintaining them is neither unproblematic nor straightforward. Enquiries into welfare tragedies regularly demonstrate the importance of comprehending processes within professional systems if the key community care policy requirements of multidisciplinary collaboration, integrated service provision and partnership between voluntary and statutory organizations are to be translated into practice and deliver an effective service.

Legislation, accompanying policy guidance and professional practice all endorse the Audit Commission's (1986) belief that collaboration is one key to effective social care. The law requires interprofessional collaboration. Health authorities and social services departments must cooperate in exercising their respective functions (NHSA 1977, section 22). Health authorities must provide, as far as is reasonable, practical and necessary, services to enable local authorities to fulfil their functions (section 26(3)). The NHS and Community Care Act 1990 (section 47(3)) reinforces this requirement. Local authorities, when assessing people's needs for community care service provision, must notify the district health authority and/or local housing authority, and invite their assistance in assessment and service provision when their help may be needed. Section 46(2) additionally requires local authorities to consult with DHAs, FHSAs, housing authorities and voluntary organizations when formulating and reviewing community care plans. The Education Act 1981 and Disabled Persons Act 1986 require collaboration between education and social services departments in relation to disabled children. Local and health authorities have joint responsibility for providing after-care to mental health service users (MHA 1983, section 117).

Policy guidance enlarges these mandates. It emphasizes the need for good working relationships based on knowledge and understanding of roles and responsibilities, and agreement on how these can be discharged (DoH 1993d). Key objectives in community care (DoH 1989a, 1990a) include promoting the development of a flourishing independent sector alongside public provision, with local authorities purchasing residential, day and domiciliary services from voluntary, not-for-profit and private agencies. Local authorities are responsible for assessing need for social care in collaboration with medical, nursing and other care agencies, with each service recognizing, respecting and using other services' contributions and responsibilities. Comparable assessment mechanisms should be created, with clarity about when health and social care needs should be assessed jointly and when one agency will contribute to another's assessment (DoH 1992a).

District health authorities must institute the care programme approach for people whose mental health needs are being addressed in the community, in collaboration with social services departments, beginning with an assessment before hospital discharge of health and social care needs. Integrated health and social care, and multidisciplinary working fundamental to its realization, is emphasized in relation to all hospital patients (SSI 1992b, c): joint objectives and targets should be established to achieve integrated continuity of care; assessment and discharge arrangements should be harmonized to ensure effective care plans. Multidisciplinary and multi-agency assessment is seen to benefit users whose specific needs are considered in relation to the whole person, with care packages tailored to the individual rather than compartmentalized into narrow agency criteria for eligibility of service (SSI 1989, 1993b). Advantages for professionals also accrue: knowledge and expertise can be shared to understand users' difficulties and to identify how best to maximize their health, welfare, choice and citizenship; and the sharing promotes awareness of roles and services.

The seamless service principle is expressed, therefore, through joint work, the mixed economy of care, and collaborative policy and procedural planning, developed locally with the purpose of removing barriers between health and social care, and of building a coherent network of local services provided by a coordinated range of professionals.

Professional practice has long recognized that teamwork in social care promotes partnership and reciprocity, and improves communication, peer support and the likelihood of providing a coherent, coordinated service involving the full range of professional skills rather than losing people's needs between services (Barclay 1982; Cambridge 1992; Knapp et al. 1992; Mann et al. 1993; Smale et al. 1993). However, while successful cooperation is undoubtedly possible, promoting partnership and reaching agreement on shared principles and methods of service provision is more complex than the legal and policy directives imply. Difficulties creating a multidisciplinary approach, threatening the principles of choice and flexibility and the development of culturally appropriate services, have surfaced in, for instance:

- premature discharge of patients without agreed plans;
- delays in care planning, and the absence of an integrated assessment of need, such that the potential, citizenship and independence of disabled people are not enhanced (SSI 1993b);
- collaborating at individual case level and interdepartmental level regarding the exchange and use of information, agreeing joint purchasing strategies and common inspection standards, promoting joint training and involving general practitioners (SSI 1992a, 1993b);
- using the Mental Illness Specific Grant initiative to provide well coordinated health and social care (SSI 1992a) or in coordinating an inter-agency approach to young disabled people (SSI 1990b);
- demarcation disputes concerning care plans, with the Department of Health (1992a) having to issue a directive to health and local authorities to work together;
- general practitioners attempting to charge social services departments for their involvement in assessment (Cervi 1993b), contradicting the 'free at the point of delivery' ethos;
- markedly differing perceptions between general practitioners and social services departments on whether agreed assessment and service protocols exist (Ivory 1993);
- local authorities failing to consult informal carers and care home owners in the drafting of community care plans.

Perhaps this should not surprise us given the number of professionals potentially required to provide flexible, sensitive and reliable community care (SSI 1992a). However, it appears complacent, when encouraging the development of inter-agency and interdepartmental policies on elder abuse (SSI 1993d), not to address those factors known from child protection experience to undermine collaboration, when the evidence questions the effectiveness of multidisciplinary collaboration. Similarly, when general practitioners are known to be uncertain about community care changes and to enjoy uneasy relationships with social services departments (Leedham and Wistow 1993), it appears curious that policy guidance merely observes that they are integral to identifying social care needs and to multidisciplinary teamworking, leaving untouched the tensions that exist. The lead role given to local authorities in social care did not command universal support in the NHS. FHSAs cannot commit individual general practitioners to particular ways of working. General practitioners, with long-established skills in assessing need and acting as advocates for their patients, can easily collide with social services departments gatekeeping limited resources and devising their own assessment schedules and criteria for service eligibility. There may also be overlap of purchaser roles for some social care services which approach the margins of health care.

Case management itself is partly a response to problems of service fragmentation, poor resource targeting and coordination, and the difficulty of interweaving informal and formal care (Levick 1992). Why, then, have the well-established systems found necessary to ensure multidisciplinary teamwork in child protection (DoH 1991i) not been reproduced for social care? Collaboration in social care will not prove any easier, nor will welfare agencies necessarily avoid their known propensity to become 'part of the problem'. Indeed, the track record of multidisciplinary teamwork remains unimpressive. There remains mistrust between agencies regarding assessment and different understandings concerning people's social care needs (DoH 1991j). Liaison between social services departments and housing authorities requires improvement, as does the working of hospital discharge arrangements (Mawhinney 1993). Private and voluntary agency providers have typically not been involved in developing community care plans, despite their knowledge of need (DoH 1992c) and ability to observe the impact of service provision. Nor have community care plans made explicit local authority proposals for involving the independent sector in day and domiciliary care (Mawhinney 1993). As service coordination has been *within* more often than between agencies (Bebbington and Charnley 1990), experience of multidisciplinary assessment and of delivering care packages is limited. Constructing workable and agreed plans with medical and housing authorities, voluntary organizations and community groups can prove difficult (Knapp *et al.* 1992), with services remaining profession-oriented rather than user-focused, and determining their involvement by their perceived capacity or, indeed, willingness to assist rather than from a structured multidisciplinary consideration of need. Summarizing, a continued need remains for collaboration and joint working, for closer integration of health and social services, to avoid duplication and to ensure coordinated contributions to social care (DoH 1993e).

Multidisciplinary collaboration is both a task to be achieved and a process to be understood and managed. Formidable obstacles lie in the path of developing a shared sense of purpose and mutual respect, of abandoning previous ways of working and looking anew at services which will realize the full potential of empowerment and partnership with users. A seamless service must engage all parts of the health and welfare system in discussion and negotiation about the principles which will inform and drive social care, and in challenging divergent ideologies, fragmentation and duplication of provision, self-interest and weak cross-agency links which continue to defeat the ideal represented in the legal and policy mandate.

Interprofessional working together: understanding the obstacles

The social care mandate

The legal and policy mandate defining the social care task is ambiguous, contradictory and incomplete. Needs, choice and resources, autonomy and paternalism, rights and risks have been juxtaposed without clarification of how any resulting confusion is to be resolved. This position reflects conflicting societal expectations about dependency, disability, older age and the role of the state and welfare agencies. Interacting with this mandate are the values of professional practice, themselves neither uniform nor consistent within and across professional groups. Sometimes these values will coincide, sometimes be in advance of and sometimes conflict with the mandate. Professionals' responses to the mandate, and the patterns of interaction thereby created, form one obstacle to collaboration.

Workers will confront key questions. What is the primary task? To what should social care aspire? What is good enough social care? Some may regard law and policy as the basis of practice; others may see their role as working to realize service users' aspirations, even where these extend practice beyond or into confrontation with approaches envisaged by law and policy. Some will prioritize professionally defined client need, others a more 'radical' agenda of wants and needs as defined by users, coupled with an understanding of how social, economic and political structures continue to disadvantage and oppress groups of people. Some will prioritize agency procedures and/or resource considerations; others a concern to avoid public scrutiny. Some will prioritize, or be asked to perform, several of these 'orientations' (Whittington 1977) simultaneously. Problems can arise, therefore, from different orientations or expectations inhabiting intra- and inter-agency systems. An illustration is when workers feel uncertain to whom or what accountability is owed when assessing need. The tensions might be obscured by distinguishing purchasers from providers but they will not be resolved so easily.

The tensions may become manifest in particular defence mechanisms or professional/agency scripts, such as when users are depersonalized and service provision takes a form of people-processing, or when moral, ethical and practice issues are reduced to questions of organizational procedures. Professionally assessed risk-taking and therapeutic work may give way to defensive practice characterized by over-assessment or a safety-first approach (Harris 1987). This may be driven by mentalism, paternalism and dominant social constructions of gender roles, race and culture, age and family roles. The professional system closes down on one definition of the problems and tasks facing social care, at times appearing to unite against users. Alternatively, the tensions may 'spill over' into disputes about perspective. How workers interpret situations will be influenced by values, training, experience, agency context and role. They may become entangled in conflicts between an individual treatment approach and practice which extends focus beyond the individual to social and economic inequalities and public attitudes which are seen as creating or exacerbating individual difficulties. Similar tangles are found in work with learning disabled people. Some professionals and carers are guided by normalization objectives; others may be concerned about users' vulnerabilities; while users themselves may feel uncertain about or insecure in community living situations (Booth et al. 1988). Unless workers can embrace perspectives other than their own, and consider the impact of competing views on the social care task, they may become 'stuck'. Relief from these tensions and 'stuckness' is sometimes sought by pulling in more professionals, a phenomenon known as triangulation (Carl and Jurkovic 1983). While designed to resolve a problematic relationship between agencies and professionals, or between them and users or carers, the triangulated professional or agency can only become 'part of the problem' because the other parties will have particular perspectives, which they will have recruited this professional or agency to endorse. This is similar to the triangulation of concepts (Chapter 4).

Besides role ambiguity and conflict, role incompatibility also frustrates collaboration. Responsibilities, whether to maintain existing services or develop new ones, are not matched by resources. Collaboration is undermined by workers not having direct control over resources (Brown and Griffiths 1993), and by uncertainties over resource availability, which create difficulties in formulating priorities, managing demanding workloads and pioneering innovation (Øvretveit 1986). How should workers respond when services which would meet needs either have not been developed or have been 'spent'? By whom and how should problems and tasks be defined? Service users may require practical and material assistance. They may benefit from the offer of psychological help. However, when confronted with escalating demands, even work overload, professional systems frequently devise gatekeeping strategies (Prodgers 1979; Addison 1982) which prioritize immediate presenting problems over deeper, more emotional issues. Agencies respond by the type of service required, such as day or residential care. This may appear to solve the problems. However, it can easily lose sight of the person and of the processes which might have created or exacerbated the situation underpinning the presenting problem. It presupposes that the problem has been identified correctly. Indeed, one danger of provider-led, problem-focused approaches is that they may overlook what takes time, skill and trust to enable users to discuss. Then, when whatever underlying the presenting problem resurfaces, services can all too easily respond with 'more of the same', a redoubling of efforts, before abandoning the user or collapsing under the strain. An approach of concerned curiosity (Cecchin 1987), exploring possibilities, feelings and anxieties, in a user-led, needs-focused enquiry may be more effective but must compete with other imperatives.

Not surprisingly then, the mandate creates anxiety and insecurity. This too can undermine collaboration. It encourages professionals and agencies to adopt a narrow focus rather than the broader view of individuals' needs promoted by policy guidance. To cope with the anxieties organizations may construct defences (Jaques 1955; Menzies 1970), such as a textbook approach which discourages the expression of emotions, dilemmas or doubts, or distancing from users by subdividing the social care task, or minimizing responsibility in assessment and decision-making in order to avoid negative reactions from users. Such defences may also be observed in individual practitioners, such as when, to cope with the anxiety of personal responsibility, workers engage in ritual task performance and/or project responsibility on to others who can then be criticized. An additional problem with these defences against anxiety is that they both generate secondary anxiety in the form of job dissatisfaction or fear of an impending crisis or new situation, and soak up vital energy in their maintenance.

Professional traditions and ideologies

The muddle generated by the social care mandate connects with different professional ideologies which may also undermine the attainment of a seamless service. Within the mixed economy of care network may reside conflicting views about acceptable levels of risk-taking, divergent views about users' interests, needs and roles (Hardy *et al.* 1993) and different understandings of needs and assessment, reflecting different ideologies or attitudes about community care (Dalley 1993). Once again, the issue is to define the primary task or parameters of social care. Left unresolved, the divergent ideologies will inspire goal and planning differences. The services envisaged by the social model of disability, for instance, to promote empowerment, citizenship and social change, will differ markedly from those inspired by an individualized medical or welfare response. Moreover, collaboration difficulties can be seen as resulting from the individualized model of service provision, coupled with minimal provision born of state reluctance to intervene (Borsay 1986).

Professional teams are highly prone to *splitting*, a process derived from personal values and attitudes, and reactions to the task, as much as from responses to the conflicting imperatives in the social care mandate. One example of this phenomenon is the masculinization of policy and practice (Grimwood and Popplestone 1993), involving the polarization of control and care, and the prioritization of skills of assessment, purchasing and inspection over those of service provision. Dividing purchasers from providers creates dangerous splits around status, power and control of the work.

One response is to agree what can be agreed, to avoid difference or conflict and to pretend that incompatible objectives do not exist (Ramon 1992). Sometimes known as *groupthink* (Janis 1972), such systems are characterized by apparent unanimity, pressures to conform, routine practice and an absence of new ideas or criticism. Goals tend to remain unquestioned, with alternatives rarely considered and evaluated. Stereotypical images of 'opposing' professional groups form the basis for the discharge of negative feelings.

Splitting and groupthink are symptoms of a closed system, fixed in its own perceptions and roles, unresponsive to ideas and different viewpoints. Such systems tend towards stagnation and disorder.

Professional space

Another source of interprofessional and inter-agency difficulty is territorial. Although policy guidance provides some indication of different roles and responsibilities in social care (DoH 1989a), problems arise when these roles, such as assessment, are common to more than one agency or professional group, and when agreement is not reached on how the various individuals and agencies may contribute to social care.

Management

Separate management hierarchies and structures create confusion and problematize communication, coordination and decision-making (CCETSW

1992a; Cornwell, 1992/3). Although well known, community care reforms have failed to incorporate a review of the structures of health and welfare provision, with the result that multidisciplinary teamwork has to be carved into existing edifices. New shapes and spaces, which facilitate clear decision-making links and coherent operational policies, have to be created in a context where differences between elected (social services committee) and appointed (FHSA, DHA) people create tensions around legitimacy, authority and status (Hardy *et al.* 1993); where some organizations can commit individual workers to particular approaches (SSD), others not (FHSA); and where different agencies have different planning and budget cycles and different resource levels, and enjoy different levels of government support. In such a context managers may feel a debt of loyalty to their own staff and become pressurized by the tasks to be met by their own agency (Ormiston and Haggard 1993).

Practice

Different agency structures and geographical boundaries also complicate the development of relationships between practitioners (Dalley 1993; Hardy *et al.* 1993; Kitzinger *et al.* 1993). Opportunities to develop teamworking, from which can develop openness, trust and a willingness to share experiences, are restricted structurally even before the consideration that much social care is provided by a network of professionals rather than a team. This is an important distinction (see Payne and Scott 1982), for groups of workers who meet rarely will encounter greater difficulty in agreeing an overall objective and experiencing the interchangeability of tasks and skills. Networks encourage distinctive as opposed to exchangeable contributions. This reinforces the legitimacy, identity and comfort which workers derive from their own professional boundaries, such that collaboration or teamwork is then perceived to threaten their domain or organizational interest (Neill 1982; Hardy *et al.* 1993). Workers may then feel little incentive to gain knowledge outside their own role and discipline (Ramon 1992), especially if questions have already been asked about the distinctiveness of their contribution. Finally, the varying degrees of contact which network members may have with users can also generate controversy: frequent contact can be viewed as over-involvement or the best way of meeting identified needs, the care management role as bringing objectivity or inappropriate distance.

Management and practice

At each organizational level collaboration can be frustrated by stereotypes, competitiveness, hostility and hidden agendas between professional groups. Mutual suspicion may arise from insecurity in one's own professionalism and contribution (Levick 1992; Corney 1993), fear of loss of status and power, role conflict and overlap (Renshaw 1988; CCETSW 1992a), such that stereotypes are maintained to preserve self-image even in the face of contradictory evidence (Preston-Shoot and Agass 1990).

Differences in power, status and experience can sabotage working together. Collaboration at practice levels may be more advanced than in higher management, such that teams may be inhibited by the lack of agency and inter-agency policies and structures to facilitate how they have agreed to work (McGrath 1993). For example, someone may only have received a simple assessment based on the local authority's tiered eligibility assessment structure, where the tiers are triggered by the initial presented need. This may not be how multidisciplinary teams wish to work together. Equally, if service providers subsequently identify this person as having more complex needs, their status and position may marginalize their power as advocates. The challenges here are the power imbalance between purchasers and providers, and the (in)flexibility of assessment procedures. If they are too rigid, they will restrict providers' autonomy to develop services as needs indicate; if too loose, they will fail to ensure effective use of scarce resources.

Positional authority, length of service and professional expertise can clash, just as imposed hierarchies – such as local authorities determining eligibility for assessment and service levels despite other professionals having assessment expertise – can generate tension. Positional authority, or norms about hierarchy (such as doctor–nurse), may run counter to skill and experience (Renshaw 1988). Concern to maximize control may complicate decision-making, which can also be affected by questions of worker gender, class and culture. The challenge here, as indeed elsewhere, is to share power in a way that empowers all staff to contribute. The challenge is to resolve the question 'who decides', to determine where authority is held. When agencies are not necessarily bound by the decisions of others, where agencies have no authority to commit the resources of other agencies to particular work plans (Øvretveit 1986) and when no umbrella organization comparable to the area child protection committee exists to resolve differences, promote agreed procedures, monitor performance and provide joint training, collaboration cannot be fully integrated into service provision.

Differences in training compound these difficulties. Not only is the practice of multidisciplinary training variable (SSI 1992d) but qualifying training pays insufficient attention to such training and to the contributions of different professional groups. Different approaches to social care are built in from the outset.

Organizations as quasi-familial groups

Collaboration is complicated further by processes derived from the interactions between workers, agencies and users. The disturbing effect of disadvantaged, oppressed and possibly distressed individuals on professionals must be better appreciated. Workers are particularly susceptible to unconscious pressure from users to take on particular feelings and act out particular roles (Preston-Shoot and Agass 1990). Left unattended this consequence of worker–user interactions can be acted out as conflict and confusion within teams and between agencies. Variously termed *mirroring, conflict by proxy* (Furniss 1983) or *system counter-transference* (Reder and Kraemer 1980), the worker/professional network reproduces and acts out psychological processes and conflicts in the user/carer network, particularly feeling states and roles. This effectively prevents the professional system working for change as it is caught in the same vicious circles as the user/carer system. It has become part of the problem.

These dynamics may be further compounded when they collide with workers' own intra- and interpersonal conflicts, that is tensions already present, generated by the social care task and/or by workers' personal experiences, but now polarized into conflict by interactions with the user/carer network. Thus, problems residing in the professional system mesh with those they must deal with in the user/carer system. Left unattended, this interplay can create a problem-maintaining cycle (Stratton et al. 1990) characterized by displacement and projection of blame, defensiveness, rigidity and/or chaos. Rather than stepping back to consider what information these interactions might provide, interactions are characterized by hopelessness, inactivity or escalating more of the same, inattention to recognizing and dealing with feelings or with the processes established by the social care task, and an absence of a structured and theoretical approach to the task.

Just as the experiences of workers and users, separately or together, may create tensions and processes which threaten to derail work, so too may the quasi-familial nature of organizations, their experiences and evolution over time, the sense made of events, the reproduction of their stories in culture and approach. Myths may have developed, beliefs which direct behaviour and which can distort communication or prevent change. Working to a formula or unquestioningly, believing that correct assessments are possible and that appropriate training can prevent tragedy are examples of myths which organizations may use to 'prevent' feared calamities and to cope with anxiety about the task. As in families, relationships may be characterized by resistance to change, resulting in a growing irrelevance of structures, roles or tasks. There may be disagreements over whether there is a problem, or how to define it, characterized by 'you change, not me' arguments. Different perspectives, such as between purchasers who seek a profile of potential providers when compiling community care plans, and providers who seek contract certainty, may compete, leaving little room for the users' voices and experiences. Like families, organizations can become locked into one solution, reproducing more of the same, such as increasingly elaborate assessment or priority schedules, or they can specify what people can and cannot do and seek to prevent discussion or change because of the feared effects this would have. They may retain behaviour which seeks to protect or to provide influence. They may act within expectations set by others in order to retain influence, for example by engaging in increasing activity to meet increasing expectations only to find a circular pattern is created whereby the expectations are maintained or escalated, resulting in increased activity to meet the required and assumed responsibilities.

As in families, boundaries and communication will also prove significant. Boundaries may be created for protection, for sub-grouping around attraction or for delineating decision-making authority. Systems where relationships are characterized by connectedness, where boundaries are sufficiently permeable to allow information exchange and change, will prove more effective than those where relationships are characterized by enmeshment (insufficient boundaries resulting in unclear decision-making authority and arrangements for information exchange, and information overload) or disengagement (boundaries too rigid, such that communication is restricted and/ or fails to reach its target). Boundaries and the communication they allow must promote flexibility and adaptability. Where they are characterized by rigidity or vagueness, the use of power to withhold or distort information exchange, or distance and disjunction between verbal communication and non-verbal behaviour, the capacity of organizations to collaborate and to evolve creatively in response to tasks will be substantially reduced.

All these obstacles can distort professional judgement, creating at worst intra- and inter-agency dangerousness (DoH 1988) and the condonation or overlooking of unacceptable practice. The barriers to partnership with the independent sector are not, therefore, just based on wariness, shortage of time and planning resources, and conflicts of interest (DoH 1992c). Accordingly, the understanding laid out above must be accompanied by tools for promoting collaboration between workers and agencies.

Keys to collaboration

As the obstacles to collaboration occur both in relation to specific pieces of work and at the structural level of agency organization, so too must tools for managing the interprofessional system embrace both individual situations and arrangements for coordinating service programmes, professional networks involving several providers from one agency and those where different agencies are involved. These tools for action must be underpinned by eight keys to collaboration, to unlocking the potential benefits for workers, users and carers of interprofessional and inter-agency cooperation.

The first key is *vision*. This is not an apostolic calling to teamwork but an analytic stance of curiosity and questioning. Variously described as being multi-minded (Grimwood and Popplestone 1993), adopting a wide angle (individuals in context) rather than telephoto (individual focus) or zoom (either individual or community) lens (Smale *et al*. 1993), or meta perspective (Selvini Palazzoli *et al*. 1978), essentially it involves moving around the professional system from the perspective of those involved rather than maintaining one fixed perspective on problem definition and problem solving. It implies standing back to monitor processes and evaluate the work of the whole professional system, including oneself and one's own agency. The purpose is to reflect on how parties see and may be seen by the system in which they are working, and to understand the complex dynamics in which they might have become enmeshed. This can open up creative dialogue and possibilities, such as when agencies conduct a 'public perception' audit to consider policies and their delivery from the public's viewpoint (Mawhinney 1993).

The second key is *power*. The imbalance of power between, say, purchasers and providers, social workers and domiciliary care workers, doctors and nurses, centred on images and perceptions of status, knowledge and training, and dimensions of race, gender and class between the individuals involved, all create unbalanced contributions, especially where these images and perceptions are internalized by those occupying 'less powerful' positions and, in the form of internalized oppression, become beliefs about the hopelessness of speaking out and about inability to contribute anything of value. Chapter 5 explored the centrality of power to questions of partnership and anti-oppressive practice, and the importance therefore of an open dialogue about power based on worker and agency recognition of power structures, worker and user perceptions of it, and how it may be used non-oppressively and anti-oppressively. Here the concern additionally is to effect change in and between organizations. For this workers and users must know where power is located and how to gain access to it. Thus, the questioning advocated as part of the first key to collaboration must include a focus on power and the extent to which the professional system is using its power, in the form of legal mandates, policy authority, resources and skills, for empowerment, for challenging oppression and for developing services *with*, not *for*, users. As already identified, decisions about provision must not be so rigid as to deny the power to develop services as needs evolve or become more clearly understood.

Exercise 7.1.   Consider the professional systems in which you work. Where does power reside in these systems? How is it used and what is the effect of its use on you, users and carers, other workers? How might they answer this question if asked? What can you or other workers do to promote the transfer of power to users? How far have agencies, separately and together, considered how users may feel empowered or oppressed by procedures and structures?

Thus, if one collaborative endeavour is to manage power in a manner which empowers colleagues and users alike, another is to manage the transfer of power to alter power differentials. This requires a willingness to cede, not just to share control. It also requires an ability to assist users to identify, value and use their power and authority.

The third key is *the introduction of difference.*

Exercise 7.2.   Take a situation with which you have struggled for some time. Consider all the approaches made to attempt progress. Are all these approaches variations of one solution, in other words more of the same?

The recognition that welfare agencies can become part of the problem suggests that it is important to intervene in the professional system if the change effort with users or carers is not to be undermined (Dungworth and Reimers 1984). This involves asking what makes it difficult for workers to abandon established ways of thinking and working, and to look anew at what services would meet users' needs. It involves keeping systems creative by introducing difference, and by creating channels for detoured conflict to be communicated and dealt with between those parts of the system where it properly resides. This commitment to 'something different' is necessary at personal, organizational and practice levels. At a personal level it is a process of unlearning and relearning, a critical scrutiny of value assumptions as a necessary foundation for considering the constructions which are placed on older age, health and (dis)ability and, therefore, the parameters which are built around social care. This 'pulling back' connects with the first key, stepping outside one's own position and viewing values, understandings and interactions between people from different perspectives.

At an organizational level it revolves around a dialogue about power, and particularly about the extent to which expert power can and should give way to learning with and facilitating users. The spotlight will be on oppressive systems, on the norms which agencies have represented. The objective will be using legislative mandates, underpinned by clear values, to inform and drive the work with and for users, rather than imposing these upon them. How do organizations perceive service users, their rights, needs and wants? What norms do standardized services express? What services would reflect an anti-oppressive approach?

At a practice level it involves promoting collective action by users, maximizing user control of processes of assessment and decision-making, and advocating clear rights for users within social care, such as resources to promote autonomy where competency is established and to promote safety for incremental risk-taking in less well-established areas, and resources to secure services which address needs as defined *by* users and which legitimate work on changing social attitudes and arrangements which restrict people's participation in society. Here the focus links with the fifth key, an emphasis on *structural* as well as personal change.

The fourth key is *creating a holding environment*. Empowering staff in the pursuit of effective anti-oppressive practice requires recognition of and dialogue about the tensions, practice dilemmas and conflicting imperatives in social care. If these are to be worked through rather than acted out, a safe and facilitating environment is required, one which encourages analysis, reflection and discussion rather than denial of the complexity. If difficulties are to be resolved collaboratively, if organizations are seriously to encourage workers to discuss the impact of agency norms and processes on themselves and users, and if workers are to be supported effectively on the task, a culture must be created where workers feel sufficiently safe to acknowledge and articulate anxiety, discomfort and disagreement. Anti-oppressive practice requires workers to put race, gender, disability and other forms of oppression on the agenda, and to demonstrate how paternalism and Eurocentricity block the needs of disabled people (Barnes 1992), women and black people. Since this may challenge one's own feelings, thoughts and actions, and will challenge established interests as encapsulated in agency policy and practice, a facilitating culture is central. Power and vision once again are keys to collaboration's potential to inspire change.

The fifth key is distinguishing between *first-* and *second-order change*. Traditionally social care law, policy guidance and practice have emphasized individualized problem-solving, leaving unchanged underlying relationships and power structures. Symptoms and tasks, rather than fundamental needs, processes and issues, are tackled. Issues which arise from the wider system are assumed to be located within individual, family or team systems and worked with as if there. When the symptoms return, or prove resistant to intervention, the system frequently responds with more of the same, for example refined procedural guidelines, rather than looking at the nature of relationships between those involved, the assumptions and norms on which these relationships are based and how intervention may have maintained or exacerbated the situation. Longer-term empowering and anti-oppressive solutions require second-order change too, based on analysis of and intervention into the context, power, culture, organizational arrangements and structural relationships which impact upon individual users and workers. This takes workers and agencies into social and political action, challenging and enabling users to challenge how they and services 'for' them have been perceived. The focus is on transactions, patterns of relationships, problems and individuals in context, with everyone in the professional network included in both analysis of what is happening and promotion of change. Thus, training for the future (DoH 1993b) and the creation of new organizational and inter-agency arrangements should focus not only on the implementation of service changes and new systems to accommodate the new arrangements (first-order change – problem solving), but also on a shifting of perspective as a basis for refocusing activity (second-order change – relationship change), for example towards partnership with users, carers and the voluntary and independent sectors.

The sixth key is *partnership*. All parts of the system must be engaged, respect must be shown for and use made of experiences, resources and contributions in individual cases and in policy formation and review. The choice of the word partnership is deliberate. It does not mean participation or consultation within preset local authority agendas, perhaps considering a draft community care plan or proposed care package. It does mean, first, all parties convening to agree how the professional system is to approach its legal and policy mandates, consulting how to work in partnership in devising an overall framework for community care. Second, it implies joint planning, for example in matching the needs and expectations of purchasers and providers in relation to contracts for services. This approach promotes mutual learning and trust, shared ownership and service relevance. It clarifies and uses difference and, through enabling the development of interprofessional and inter-agency agreements about aims, principles and procedures (Hardy *et al.* 1993; Leedham and Wistow 1993), it improves outcomes for users.

The seventh key is *visibility*. Developing joint mechanisms for achieving integrated care, and for monitoring and reviewing performance and outcome of objectives (SSI 1992c), requires commitment: to building new relationships and organizational structures, to dealing with disagreement and difference openly, to sharing information and professional territories. The creation and sustaining of this approach will be facilitated by its being visible (Ormiston and Haggard 1993): in joint events, such as planning days to engage in or review joint work, or identify and use resources within the system; in action research; in training courses, linked to policy development, coordinated and planned by an inter-agency group; in publicity about achievements; in delegation to managers and workers of decision-making autonomy sufficient to progress work. The idea of a health and social care 'passport', a user-held record (Henwood 1993), not only provides users with a greater sense of personal control but also, in merging records of assessments, plans, actions by those involved and outcomes, demonstrates evidence of change from traditional practice to a shared philosophy and approach to collating information and enabling users to express their needs or exercise their rights in a coordinated service. Scepticism, resistance and cynicism about community care changes generally, and multidisciplinary collaboration, particularly, will not be overcome by encouragement alone. It requires managerial support and a clear demonstration of commitment and possibilities.

The final key to collaboration is *the distinction between task and process*. The erratic track record of multidisciplinary collaboration suggests some attention to processes to achieve the task. Guidance abounds:

- overarching values, to provide direction and standards, and to avoid stereotyping;
- clarity of purpose and structure (Onyett 1992; Hardy *et al.* 1993), each informed by a comprehensive survey of needs;
- robust and coherent management arrangements (Hardy *et al.* 1993);
- defining the function of resources such as residential care (Neill 1982) and focusing on objectives of resourcing rather than just on the resources available;
- team control over deployment of services and resources (Knapp *et al.* 1992; McGrath 1993);
- team coordinators accepted by all the professions involved (McGrath 1993);
- single transferable procedures for assessment, one entry point via different services (DoH 1991c);
- flexible service models, neither so loose as to be chaotic and unstructured, nor so rigid as to restrict autonomy and workers' abilities to develop and implement expertise.

Exercise 7.3.   Consider the agency within which you work. To what extent has this agency, separately or in partnership with others, clearly distinguished and publicized the values which inform practice, the aims of social care, the objectives which are derived from service aims, priorities and methods for achieving and reviewing the objectives?

Within an overarching framework for the task, agencies must consider the collaborative structures and strategies needed to meet the legal mandate to coordinate services. This requires clarity about roles and responsibilities. Thus negotiation and agreement is required on:

- who will coordinate, at what organizational level, the interface with other agencies, monitoring individual cases, team functioning and services, with clarity about how this will inform planning, resourcing and objective setting;

- what type of teams or networks are required for policy planning and review, for service delivery to user groups. This relates to membership, supervision and management of teams, where different models (Øvretveit 1986; Onyett 1992) are possible;
- how workloads will be managed to avoid overload and to ensure effective targeting of services based on assessment of need and priority decisions (Orme and Glastonbury 1993);
- what is profession-specific, on the basis of how each profession perceives and approaches its tasks, what overlaps different professions and may be undertaken variously, such as assessment, and what is common to different professions, i.e. not profession-specific (Øvretveit 1986);
- communication based on need rather than position (Biggs 1990);
- how roles will be allocated and disputes resolved.

Exercise 7.4.   In relation to situations you are working in, are you clear where responsibility lies for decisions about approach, for coordinating contributions, for deciding workload management and priority issues? Is there clarity about the personnel and skill resources required, and about how to resolve questions of overlap and gaps in knowledge and skills?

Thus, when you are 'troubleshooting', teamwork problems may reside in the task: unrealistic goals; inadequate resources of time, services and/or skills available to team members; blocks in other systems. Equally, problems may arise from conflictual relationships, from doubts about investing in goals, from group processes.

Exercise 7.5.   Do the teams considered in the previous exercise have structures which facilitate encouragement, mediation, clarification of and reflection on process? What strengths and themes, alliances and exclusions, and communication patterns do you observe? What happens to communication within the system and between systems? What does this suggest?

This highlights the importance of maintenance work (Kitzinger *et al.* 1993) in negotiating and sustaining relationships, recognizing that team development is marked by stages (Preston-Shoot 1987), with trust, experimentation with different ways of working, expression of difference and flexible working patterns requiring groupwork skills to develop.

Teamworking interventions

Several tools are useful for practitioners and teams seeking to implement the keys to collaboration and manage the obstacles in the interprofessional system. The first, *hypothesizing*, centres on key questions.

- What is the problem?
- Why is it a problem now?
- Where is the problem?
- What might be the meaning, function or purpose of the problem?

Where the 'stuckness' resides in the interaction between the professional system and the user/carer/family system, additional questions (Dimmock and Dungworth 1983; Dungworth and Reimers 1984; Stratton *et al.* 1990) help to formulate an effective intervention.

- What role is being pressed on the team and why?
- Is this role appropriate to accept?
- With whom does the team need to clarify its role?
- How do people view the interactions, their position in this system and the position of others?
- Who believes there are (what) problems? Is there a problem definition which agencies are working on? Is this shared with the user/carer/family system?

Essentially, hypotheses are stories, meta perspectives about processes and how these are enacted within and between systems. They help to clarify what is happening and, thereby, to give purpose and direction to the change effort. If unclear values are driving the work, questions of rights and risks may need to be debated. If misconceptions exist about what different professionals can and should do, stereotypical beliefs and models of understanding social care tasks may need to be shared. If the work is triggering anxiety and this is affecting decision-making, support may have to be sought.

The second tool is *naming*, setting out this understanding in a manner which values people's contribution where possible since they will find it more difficult to contemplate difference and change if they feel blamed. Positive reframes may then be followed with questions about what the system could do more effectively in this or similar situations. This requires a third tool, *convening the system*. This enables observation of how system members interact, the position people adopt. This can be useful in exploring the position of the referring person in the system referred (Selvini Palazzoli *et al.* 1980; Preston-Shoot and Agass 1990), the nature of relationships and whether another agency or professional is being triangulated (Carl and Jurkovic 1983) to resolve a problematic relationship. It may enable work done by one part of the professional system to be observed by others, thereby avoiding duplication or being drawn into problem sequences (Benbow *et al.* 1990; Bowman and Jeffcoat 1990). Convening the system also helps to sustain working together, to share perspectives which help to define what intervention to make, and to explore openly differences in goals. The nature of relationships and communication can be illustrated by use of sculpting, geneograms and eco-maps (Stratton *et al.* 1990) to map: significant strong, weak and/or conflictual relationships; significant events; how such relationships and events have been carried subsequently into organizational life; how structures and relationships may block or distort communication; boundaries, roles, feelings and the perceptions of system members about these.

Convening the system helps to avoid covert agendas and relates the worker–user encounter to the systems which underpin it. It engages the professional system in problem clarification and resolution, and reduces the likelihood of acting out disagreements, of splitting into 'good and bad' agencies, and enmeshment in one person's problem definition (Pottle 1984; Dungworth 1988; Stratton *et al.* 1990). The system to convene should depend on need, not position, and may include family, friends and local community figures who provide support (Pottle 1984).

The fourth tool is *hunting the latitude* (Stratton *et al.* 1990), searching for those areas where system members have room for manoeuvre, alternative ways of understanding and tackling a problem. It involves acknowledging the common tendency to use favourite approaches, and suspending 'bias' to ensure that possibilities are not neglected (Smale *et al.* 1993). One such latitude lies in reducing restraining forces rather than increasing driving forces, since the latter will increase anxiety and tension (De Board 1978). Another is asking what decisions are non-negotiable, usual and possible, identifying which are least acceptable and why, and by a process of such elimination finding the decision people feel least anxious about (O'Brian and Bruggen 1985). Negotiations can also be freed by recognizing that, while mutuality or complete agreement on objectives and methods of achieving them might be desirable, reciprocity, where exploration leads to narrowing differences and a balance of agreement which outweighs disagreement, might be a useful starting point, parties agreeing to work on each other's objectives. A consultant, someone outside the system, may provide a different perspective (Dare *et al.* 1990), expanding the team's imagination by generating fresh ideas about difficulties, the processes which maintain or aggravate them and the work required to overcome them. A consultant can help teams to track processes within the system, and between it and other systems, and how these processes might reflect the internal and interpersonal processes in the user/carer/family system (Preston-Shoot and Agass 1990).

Conclusion

The inbuilt fragmentation between purchasing and providing, health and social care, local authorities and the independent and voluntary sectors makes a seamless service a difficult goal to achieve. The systems approach, on which this chapter is based, adds a useful dimension to understanding and intervening in interprofessional and inter-agency systems. It complements other essential competencies for multidisciplinary work in social care: identifying the parts of and relationships between agencies; understanding the different perspectives of other professionals, including the values, knowledge and skills each offer; being able to use knowledge from other professionals while being clear regarding one's own perspective (Biggs and Weinstein 1991).

8 Managing the personal experience of work

Two themes have permeated this book: the complexity of social care, the dilemmas, challenges and possibilities facing those seeking to provide quality services; and empowerment of practitioners and managers to enable them to respond to the challenges and realize the potential of empowering practice. Working with people, and the complexity of providing care, frequently involves anxiety, risk and dilemma management, choices between different valued courses of action and complicated decisions about whether and how to intervene. Practitioners and managers must act on judgements of risk and need, knowing that they cannot eliminate doubt, within a context of stretched resources. They will not always satisfy everyone involved. They may struggle with how to reconcile their professional values and training, their concepts of good practice, with agency-based realities. This work is stressful.

Stress has more commonly been associated with child protection work than with social care, betraying assumptions about the common-sense nature and basis of providing care. Child protection work does generate substantial stress, to which practitioners and their managers must respond if they are to perform their roles and responsibilities effectively. However, little is known about stress in social care, despite the high demands which such work places upon staff coping with challenging behaviour and tasks in a context of inadequate time, resources, training and management support (Knapp *et al.* 1992); despite recognition of the need to provide support systems for staff, for instance when working with elder abuse (Penhale 1993; SSI 1993d) or within the sometimes highly charged, difficult and demanding environments of residential care or day centres (Bernard *et al.* 1988; Brown 1990).

Work-related stress is associated with anxiety, depression and burn-out (Menzies 1970; Cooper and Marshall 1978; Payne and Firth-Cozens 1987;

Gibson *et al.* 1989; Jones *et al.* 1991; Sutherland and Cooper 1992); with poor organizational performance, reflected in low morale, absenteeism, staff turnover and poor service quality (Pines and Maslach 1980); and with management styles (Pottage and Evans 1992) where the caring strand of management has been neglected in community care reforms (Grimwood and Popplestone 1993) and managers are inadequately trained, resourced and supported for the tasks and responsibilities they must carry out and for the rate and degree of change they must manage (King 1991; Brindle 1992; Cohen 1992).

When pressure on individuals and organizations exceeds their available resources and creates stress, this seriously impedes work performance. Experiences of working with disturbing situations, with difficult and challenging people, and the susceptibility of the professional system to interprofessional conflict illustrate how effective practice can give way to professional defensiveness and dangerousness at both personal and inter-organizational levels. A corruption of care (Wardhaugh and Wilding 1993) can result from the intense emotional pressure to which practitioners may be subjected and the organizational and resource context in which work takes place. Individuals are regularly castigated for the outcomes of critical incidents but dangerousness and stress are not simply individual phenomena. Stress levels and effects are affected by the interaction between demands and the internal and external resources within the system upon which people may call (Wiener 1989; J. Williams 1991).

Stress, therefore, is a key theme for empowering practice in social care. Practitioners and managers must consider how to create a safe environment where the personal experience of work can actively be addressed without individuals being pathologized or perceived as inadequate. This requires frameworks for understanding and action, to enable organizations and workers to respond creatively to the anxieties created by their tasks, and to acquire and maintain skills and processes for managing the personal experience of work.

Definitions and principles

Stress results when individuals experience demands as exceeding their available resources, and as pushing them beyond physical and/or psychological stability (Cummings and Cooper 1979; Gardener 1988). This interactive definition focuses on external adversity and pressures, on the internal effects of those pressures and on factors internal to individuals which influence how work is experienced. It focuses attention on the interaction between the internal and external; between individuals and their organizational and social context; between the demands and the resources available to moderate them. The definition implies that when stress is controlled, when demands and resources are balanced, it can enhance performance. Without such balance it may become dysfunctional, characterized by increased activity but reduced performance, and by physical symptoms, anxiety or work avoidance. Left unattended, stress can escalate to 'paralysis' (Baker 1986), involving disturbed behaviour and difficulties in, or non-performance of, work.

This definition generates some key principles to guide individuals and organizations in understanding the sources of stress and devising strategies for its management (Preston-Shoot and Braye 1991). The first is that work inevitably involves personal, emotional experiences which can provoke anxiety. These experiences may trigger personal issues and/or professional dilemmas and doubts, which workers should examine and share in order to remain effective. The second principle is that strategies will involve group and organizational problem-solving alongside personal adjustment. To deal effectively with stress requires both self-analysis and political action (Addison 1982) because stress originates not just from an individual's own emotions, reactions and behaviour, but also from the context and structures of employing organizations and from the competing views of the various stakeholders in social care services. In other words, the sources of stress are just as likely to reside in how work is organized as in workers themselves and, therefore, strategies must be concerned with individual workers and with organization development and change (Murgatroyd 1992).

To be useful, these strategies must offer a framework for understanding the sources of stress and the factors that can make changing working practices difficult. They must focus on the interaction and interconnectedness between individuals, organizations and their social context, and enable practitioners and managers to find positive, practical ways forward. They must be easy to use within busy work schedules, and become part of the work culture at every level of an organization, used proactively rather than reactively in response to individual crisis. Finally, they should be capable of appraisal in terms of the difference they make over time.

Sources of stress in social care services

Exercise 8.1.   Identify the sources of stress which (may) appear when you work (a) in your organization, (b) with service users and their families, (c) with colleagues, (d) with multi-agency systems. Identify the key components of your job and pinpoint (a) what you feel anxious about and when, (b) what you find it hardest to cope with, (c) how you cope with what you have pinpointed.

Studies of stress pinpoint interactions with service users: the emotional effects of working with vulnerable or disturbing people, of anticipating or encountering violence or aggression, or of having offers of help refused; and the experience of the organizational structure for, and the context of, the work. A pervading sense of powerlessness appears: powerlessness to influence how jobs are defined, to influence externally imposed change, to manage competing and conflicting demands, to have sufficient resources to complete the work safely and effectively and to ensure adequate training and supervision. Individuals and organizations alike must address six key areas.

Work-related stresses

The legal framework is one source of stress (Davies and Brandon 1988; Jones *et al.* 1991; Bennett *et al.* 1993). This should not surprise us. The volume and complexity of law which impinges upon social care, the tensions and dilemmas contained within it and government guidance, and the sometimes uneasy juxtaposition between professional values and legislative intentions all influence how the legal framework is viewed. The complexity, inexplicitness and inconsistencies within the legal framework create uncertainty about whether, how and when to act. The law performs a range of social functions and is influenced by competing factors: political ideology; social norms; values and assumptions about people, relationships and society; and different approaches to need, risk, choice and partnership (Braye and Preston-Shoot 1992a). Consequently, social care professionals face conflicting imperatives, for instance between needs and rights, or autonomy and protection, under which the pursuit of one set of principles forces the abandonment of others, or leaves professionals holding the tension of a difficult middle ground. Practitioners are also confronted by practice dilemmas, where, again, rigid adherence to one side of the equation will mean neglecting its opposite, and where often there will be no 'right answer' about the best course of action (see Figure 8.1).

A further source of stress is role conflict. The themes of partnership, choice, empowerment and needs-led assessments, as cornerstones of service delivery, are capable of different interpretations and conflict with the emphasis on available resources. Workers find their notions of good practice compromised by the service realities they encounter. Their assessments are devalued or rendered less effective by resource scarcity and agency reluctance to identify need clearly because of the consequent legal obligation to provide services to meet it.

Another feature is role uncertainty or role ambiguity. Not only do medical and social models of, say, disability lead to fundamentally different approaches to social care, but definitions of practice competence (CCETSW 1991b) are contradictory. Workers must counteract oppression, mobilize users' rights and promote choice, yet act within organizational and legal structures which users experience as oppressive. While working in partnership, practitioners must adhere to organizational decision-making processes which limit user participation and, on occasion, make decisions for users. The practice dilemmas already referred to emanate from contradictory public and political expectations, arising from an absence of consensus on key questions: when protection of vulnerable people (risk factors) must assume paramountcy over rights (self-determination); when an ethical duty of care must be expressed in terms of statutory control; how agencies should intervene to protect older people from abuse and (self-)neglect. The central challenge for empowering social care is how anti-discriminatory and anti-oppressive practice can be implemented in agency contexts where statutory duties and regulations predominate.

Thus, stress may arise from:

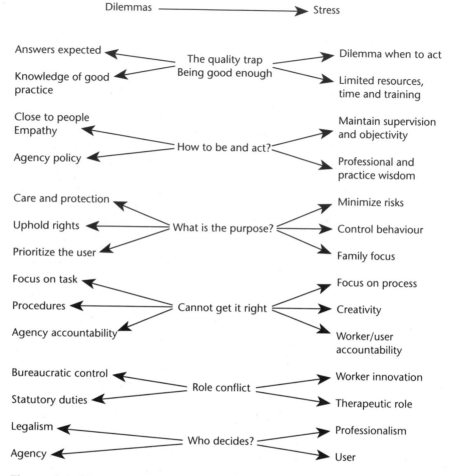

Figure 8.1 Managing the personal experience of social care practice.
Source: Preston-Shoot and Braye (1991).

- competing versions of the task;
- failure to address the anxiety and anger that can result when new ways of working are introduced, which implicitly question what has been done previously (CCETSW 1992a);
- failure to provide resources such as day support, education and leisure services, and employment opportunities for users, and underestimation of users' needs for staff support and, therefore, the staffing levels and flexible working arrangements required (Knapp *et al.* 1992);
- underestimation of the degree of control in social care (Grimwood and Popplestone 1993) and failure to address the power imbalance between users and practitioners;
- ignoring the dangers which can arise when practitioners concentrate on the most difficult situations while themselves being accorded low status

(Wardhaugh and Wilding 1993) – of concern here are the variable and unsocial hours, exploitative employment contracts, absence of a career structure, restricted employment choices and security, low wages and limited supervision and training which characterize some social care jobs (SSI 1992a; Cornwell 1992/3).

Service-user-related stresses

Working in situations of material and/or emotional deprivation, disturbed and disturbing behaviour, unmet needs and vulnerability is stressful. So too is witnessing distress or continued deterioration and communication difficulty with users, where practitioners remain uncertain whether they are valued (Rogers 1990). There is the challenge of finding the line between a positive professional relationship and friendship, and the tendency for agencies to underestimate the psychological and emotional effects of support work (Knapp et al. 1992). Brown (1990) refers to the demands of coping with authority and control, conflict, intimacy and confidentiality when working in residential and day care settings. Maintaining key professional values, such as openness and honesty, is not always straightforward. Practice will evoke strong feelings and draining emotions (Preston-Shoot and Agass 1990) which, whether obvious or more subtle, can be telling in their effects, such that retaining a professional role becomes stressful and difficult if the feelings and reactions are not managed constructively.

Individual-related stresses

Workers regularly report that training ill-equips them for practice, and that supervision, if available at all, focuses on agency accountability at the expense of staff support and development. They express concerns about the implications of changes (Rogers 1990; SSI 1992c), feeling that their knowledge and skills as providers are undervalued or insufficient in the emphasis now placed on care planning and organization of services. Where reforms have required role change, stress arises from uncertainty or acute self-consciousness, from uncertain competence in new tasks. Not unnaturally, individuals are concerned about whether their training and experience will be appropriate for the demands of social care practice.

The emphasis here is also on self-expectations and needs, on personal experiences and triggers, especially when these become hooked into external demands. Woolfe (1992) encourages workers to concentrate on stress arising 'from me'. People generate stress for themselves, arising from a desire to be loved, to receive recognition or to satisfy unrealistic expectations. These unmet needs or reactions, often derived from life experience and scripts internalized in childhood, can be reactivated by and acted out in work (Malan 1979; Bacon 1988; Carr 1989). Self-awareness is highly important, therefore. Otherwise work may become blocked and less effective because workers are unable to maintain appropriate boundaries between themselves and their work or other people, or are responding inappropriately to the work, doing either too much or too little, avoiding action or pursuing one approach to the exclusion of others, because of their own needs (Gardener 1988; Preston-Shoot and Agass 1990).

Organization-related stresses

Stress may arise from perceived distance between managers and practitioners, and from managerial failure to demonstrate understanding of pressures upon staff and to provide support and feedback to meet workers' emotional needs. This may result in workers feeling undervalued and may be connected to the corruption of care found in residential settings. The different values and priorities for service delivery that practitioners and managers may hold can generate tension. However, with partnership a key tenet of empowering practice in social care, a major source of stress arises from workers believing that they are not regarded as partners by their managers. Involving practitioners in decisions affecting them is central to an effective organization. However, they often report little knowledge or involvement in community care implementation, uncertainty about future work and exclusion from policy development and decision-making about organizational change (SSI 1992b). Organizational cultures have remained hierarchical rather than partnership-centred. Information and status are used as power, roles are possessively guarded and boundaries rigidly maintained.

The organization of the work may generate stress. Case managers have reported that stress arises from the absence of a peer reference group (Levick 1992). Individual caseloads, with restricted opportunities for co-working or peer consultation, and shift systems in residential care which limit openings for teamwork and development, are associated with stress. So too are high demand, such as required speed in decision-making, accompanied by low autonomy whereby individual action is restricted (Bennett et al. 1993), and working in organizations where staff development and training policies are not directly linked to and informed by operational requirements and worker need.

A third element is system stress (Murgatroyd 1992). Chapter 7 explored the difficulties which can arise in the interprofessional system to derail purposeful work. How members within organizations and multiprofessional systems relate to each other and how organizations meet the demands generated by the work and its context will affect stress levels. Thus, Brown (1990) refers to relationships becoming distorted by organizational and psychological pressures such as power, envy, comparison and competitiveness; Wardhaugh and Wilding (1993) to the context producing inward-looking organizations which block out new ideas and critical appraisal of task and process issues, adopting routinized practices which can become less effective, and even dangerous. Jones and Novak (1993) similarly identify the dangers of agency defensiveness, where ethical and effective practice is abandoned in favour of agency protection. Different priorities, values or approaches to social care practice, coupled with poor communication channels within and between organizations, may contribute to stress, as can subgroupings and unrealistic, imposed workloads.

Race-related stresses

Racism remains prevalent in welfare organizations and affects practitioners and users alike. White power and privilege in relationships with black people, together with normative and stereotypical assumptions, still underpin law and practice, and perpetuate the provision of inappropriate services (Dutt 1990). Indeed, compliance by local authorities with duties to promote equality of opportunity and the provision of non-discriminatory services (section 71, RRA 1976) remains exceedingly disappointing. There are few anti-racist policies and practices which are comprehensive and promote access to services that are responsive to needs (SSI 1992a). If services are still dominated by white norms, it also remains true that black people fare badly in employment (Mihill 1991) and face the added stress of having to work in white organizations (Grandison 1992).

Gender-related stresses

Employment law reinforces gender ideology and has made little impact on women's employment position (Braye and Preston-Shoot 1992a) and social welfare organizations maintain the gendering of society (Phillipson 1992), both resulting from and perpetuating a devaluing of women's skills and a general neglect of career planning, management development and training for women. Women are offered opportunities in individualistic and haphazard ways without any systematic assessment of their needs (SSI 1992e). This has coincided with a devaluing of caring roles generally, and of the caring strand of management (Grimwood and Popplestone 1993), and an increasing emphasis on identifying management and practice with masculine skills. Women commonly encounter both overt and covert sexism at work, and frequently work in situations which are potentially abusive, and even dangerous.

Counterproductive responses

These stresses may lead to individuals experiencing physical illness, depression or insomnia, and reducing social contacts. Withdrawal from colleagues, exhaustion, apathy, difficulty in concentrating, fear of decision-making and insatiable demands for support may also arise. Various defences may be used: denial, internalization (it's all my fault) or externalization (it's all their fault) (Gardener 1988); reaction formation, where hostility is translated into placatory attitudes; and displacement, where anger is vented on innocent people. These defences may temporarily reduce anxiety but the source remains untouched. As defences also deplete resources, the 'solution' can become part of the problem, with further loss of effectiveness. Defences, while they are understandable responses, ultimately render change more difficult if they are not addressed.

Organizations can also react defensively against anxiety. Different ideologies of need, such as economics, moral terminology and eligibility criteria

(Smith and Harris 1972), may be used to reduce user demands and cope with the volume of tasks. Office arrangements and depersonalization, where people are referred to by categories, may distance users from practitioners and practitioners from managers. Bureaucratic rigidity, with tight and defensive procedures, is designed to minimize risk and eliminate error. What is absent is a dialogue about the contradictory requirements asked of welfare agencies. These individual and organizational defences can result in vicious circles (Preston-Shoot and Agass 1990; Preston-Shoot and Braye 1991). They may also be depicted as downward spirals. Tension created by the work context results in withdrawal, which creates isolation. This generates fear, which increases the tension experienced, and so on. Alternatively, tension may result in increased activity and working harder. Maintaining this level of activity results in reduced effectiveness, which exacerbates the tension and further increases activity. If not interrupted, this spiral will cause burnout. If uninterrupted, defences must be escalated to retain the same desired effect of reducing stress and containing anxiety, to which is added the recognition of reduced work satisfaction inherent in this situation and anxiety, not only about work but also about having to maintain these defences.

Strategies for managing stress

Exercise 8.2.   Identify what helps you to manage the stresses of your job. Review your practice and experience of work, and identify (a) what empowers you and disempowers you in your work, (b) what your managers could do to help you in your work and (c) what you might change to help you at work.

This chapter's interactive definition of stress prompts organizational, group and individual strategies. These are likely to include personal resources and qualities, such as a sense of humour and positive attitudes of mind, but also the commitment of managers to availability and supportiveness, to supervision and a willingness to structure work with staff needs in mind. Fundamental is the creation of an organizational culture which provides safety for the expression of concerns and feelings, as part of a wider commitment to manage power, to manage staff and to manage the task in a way that empowers those involved in social care to practise.

Organizational strategies

The sources of stress indicate the broad areas for managers where strategies are required. To ensure their relevance, however, information is needed about how *this* organization and its members perceive and experience the work. This requires a *stress audit*, the first strategy, which is reviewed periodically, on the basis of which the organization develops an *action plan*, the second strategy, to manage the anxiety and stress evoked by the work.

A stress audit, using questionnaires and interviews, provides an analysis of the main sources of stress as experienced by staff. People at different

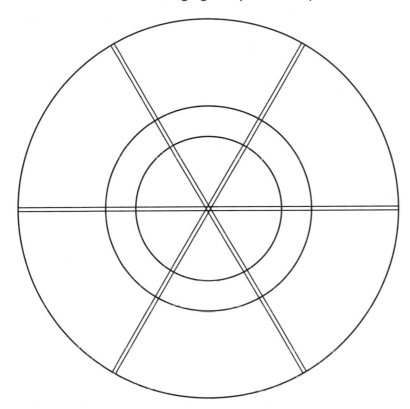

Figure 8.2 Managing the personal experience of work.

locations in the organization will identify both similar and different sources of stress, and action perceived as likely to be beneficial. The audit's results should be analysed in partnership with staff and, as sources of stress to be managed, form the first stage of the action plan (see Figure 8.2).

The segments of the innermost circle in Figure 8.2 will each contain one issue or problem, one source of stress. The next circle will contain information on its severity or frequency, and what efforts have been made previously to manage it. The organization then engages in consultation about possible approaches to address the identified issues or sources of stress. Agreed approaches are described in the outermost circle. They should include who will be involved, how and when, and review arrangements. This process promotes connectedness in an organization (Murgatroyd 1992), creating a culture of partnership where staff have a sense of belonging. In planning how to tackle issues, a useful approach is to 'hunt the latitude', to search for those areas where individually and collectively there is room for manoeuvre (Stratton et al. 1990). This search for alternative ways of understanding and tackling problems requires a safe atmosphere which encourages playfulness with ideas, investing in the strengths and perspectives that people bring. Action planning attempts to devise structural solutions to problems and stressors. Implementation of action plans will require the commitment of those with power and authority in the organization (J. Williams 1991), dialogue between managers and practitioners, and the engagement of key people in the change process. This approach opens up communication within an organization.

The third organizational strategy focuses on *staff care practices*. Pursuant to the organization's recognition and acceptance of the inevitability of stress is the provision, independent of line management, of confidential counselling services (J. Williams 1991). However, these services remain an exception rather than the rule. Other staff care practices include regular supervision, which focuses, beyond monitoring and discussion of tasks to meet agency accountability, on the work's impact on the supervisee and the interactions between the supervisee and the users with whom she or he works; on providing feedback and identifying training needs; on induction programmes, staff appraisal and personal development planning (Preston-Shoot 1991). This provides another means for validating an individual's strengths and for pin-pointing areas for development, both of which may be addressed through supervision and training which aims to develop both stress management and work-based skills.

One note of caution must be sounded. The sources of stress identified above, and the practice dilemmas highlighted throughout this book, represent difficulties within the social care task and an absence of consensus about how the task should be understood. Training and staff development, as we warned in Chapter 3, can very easily be recruited to 'solve' this problem. They cannot solve competing versions of the task, nor such organizational pressures as resource shortage. Nor should they be used solely as a remedial provision for individuals. Training should be broader than a focus on skill development, to include a staff and organizational development approach, where agency policies and strategies are connected directly to individual and group learning needs. Equally, knowledge and skills from training will wither if not linked to an empowering agency culture containing, *inter alia*, supervision, teamwork and appraisal.

The fourth organizational strategy focuses on *interactions between people*, whether within teams or within multidisciplinary, multi-agency working groups. As Chapter 7 illustrated, group and team processes can reflect dynamics between practitioners and users, or be locations where anxiety is acted out rather than contained. Convening these systems, through meetings, case discussion and support groups, and team building or away-day events, is useful for keeping channels of communication open, for breaking down isolation within and between teams, for sharing anxiety and discussing uncertainty, for identifying individual resources and maximizing their use in teams or groups, and for facilitating coordination between teams or groups and agencies. This helps to prevent isolation and to promote a coherent service.

The fifth organizational strategy revolves around *organization of work*. With role ambiguity and role conflict featuring as sources of stress, clarification of expectations and duties within and between jobs is essential. Providing clearer role definition is one means of reducing stress (King 1991), and involves the agency in defining the mandates it is required by law to meet and those which it will empower practitioners to work within. This includes support to workers to develop partnership and anti-oppressive practice and, in promoting such practices as normalization, the provision of structured risk-taking procedures.

If definition of the organization's value base and policies is one component here, another is building appropriate responses to anxiety, overload and isolation by giving thought to job design and by considering what effects work may have. Variety within work and responsibility for whole rather than just pieces of work (Makin et al. 1989) promote satisfaction. Within social care, the opportunity to respond flexibly to user need, to move beyond narrow considerations of service eligibility in assessment towards a more holistic and problem focused approach, has been welcomed (Levick 1992). The building in of mechanisms for responding to difficult situations with users, such as possible violence, together with the use of debriefing groups after critical incidents to talk through experiences and feelings, to identify legal and practice issues and to pinpoint practitioners' strengths, again promotes work satisfaction. Managed and realistic workloads are also central, with unrealistic demands undermining staff morale and threatening quality of provision (Knapp et al. 1992). The ability of services and practitioners to maintain the quality of life enjoyed by users, and to provide flexible services to prevent unnecessary admission to residential care, will be undermined by resource constraint, unclear priorities, inadequate assessment and review procedures and work overload, with a consequent effect on staff morale.

A career and advancement policy is also important. Residential workers, part-time staff and domiciliary care staff are examples of groups of workers who often feel that they are disadvantaged in career terms, afforded low status and overlooked in terms of training, contracts of employment and the effects of working hours or shifts on their physical health and emotional or interpersonal well-being. Greater flexibility in work arrangements would benefit morale, as would equality of opportunity with full-time and/or higher status colleagues.

The sixth organizational strategy refers to *workplace culture*: attention not just to task but also to process, creating a culture of caring and support which fosters creativity and growth. This chapter has already referred to the importance of valuing staff, of involving them in policy formation and decision-making, of creating a sense of partnership and belonging. It has emphasized the importance to morale and satisfaction of recognizing organizational and individual racism and sexism, and creating a safe environment where these, besides stress more generally, may be raised without fear of being pathologized. Racial and sexual harassment policies and equal opportunities within employment will feature here. Equally, with practitioners aware of the political dimension which underpins their work, an agency willingness to discuss this openly, especially its effects on, and how to safeguard and promote, the professional value base, may help to counteract the cynicism, scepticism and disillusionment which so often feature among workers. For they are often left to struggle alone with the conflict within and between complex and confused legal mandates and professional commitments to anti-discriminatory and anti-oppressive practice, to a needs-based service which focuses beyond individuals and on to the context in which they live, and which targets social and structural as well as individual change. The pressure to accommodate to legislative changes and government philosophy can easily lead to neglect of purposes inspired by the professional value base and to unquestioning practice, unless space for debate is created.

Individual strategies

Individual practitioners, in completing Exercise 8.2, will have undertaken a *stress audit* of the factors which facilitate and hinder their work. If this exercise is a tool for understanding the work context and oneself, for reflection and for stepping outside oneself in order to release creative energy for tackling problems, then the first tool for action is to translate the results into the *individual action plan*. The key choice facing practitioners when they consider their response to stress is whether to employ accommodation strategies, to contain and manage anxiety and stress, or whether to adopt change strategies. Examples of the former include support groups and supervision; of the latter, personal therapy, supervision and political action. The crucial point is that in failing to address the issues underlying stress, practitioners and managers risk their coping mechanisms becoming part of the problem, not the hoped-for solution (Woolfe 1992). There is no correct strategy to follow. Much will depend on personal preference and the situations in which people find themselves. The following strategies should be seen, therefore, as possibilities.

Interacting within organizational structures

There are five elements here. The first is avoiding self-sacrifice by recognizing the limits of responsibility and questioning whether personal objectives are realistic within the resources available. Developing individual and team approaches to saying no, to managing boundaries, coupled with identifying and communicating what is needed to work effectively, are pertinent here. The second is examining roles, searching particularly for what practitioners are experiencing or would rather not see. Relevant questions here include asking what roles people, both users and members of the professional system, are asking workers to play.

The third element is challenging the system when you are invited to overturn or abandon professional judgement, that is when you are invited to make decisions other than on the basis of professional knowledge, skills and values. Being invited to compromise needs-led assessments is an obvious example here. Fourth, practitioners may insist on supervision, and on debriefing after significant events. Agency systems should acknowledge the positive effects of praise, recognition and feedback, and focus on how the working environment could be improved. Finally, workers may look for themes and issues arising from work with individual cases, and introduce work based on these themes and issues into the agency. Such networking can be a powerful form of support and learning, can promote action for change by users and practitioners, and can provide the agency with information for planning future service provision.

Individual practice strategies

Strategies here include particular practice skills. Incorporating planning and reflecting time, what Woolfe (1992) calls anticipatory coping, helps practitioners to identify and respond to the issues which confront them in particular situations, and to express uncertainty when it is felt. So does cultivating a meta position or supervisory viewpoint (Casement 1985), whereby individuals critically appraise their goals and work for clarity, priorities and timescales, and engage in personal learning reviews to identify strengths, resources and staff development needs. The emphasis here is on skills of analysis. This may be through looking for the not so obvious, since anxiety can often be unravelled by exploration of contexts, causal links and hidden meanings. It may be through considering what can be changed in the agency, team and/or personal practice, what positive reframes can be found for what is experienced in the team, agency and/or work, and what interventions can be made. Room for innovative responses may also arise from sharing feelings, as a black worker, as a woman, as a domiciliary carer (Grandison 1992), identifying what and who can help, how and when.

Individual process

Strategies here focus on personal awareness. The emphasis is on individuals identifying from where particular processes, such as the need to be helpful or feelings of defensiveness and anxiety, might originate: what might be triggering such processes, what emotions the work evokes and what support systems are available for use.

Antidotes

The strategies here enable a balance to be found between work and non-work. Social activities, humour, physical exercise – whatever individuals enjoy doing to unwind healthily – are important for incorporation into a stress management approach.

Conclusion

All these strategies, individual and organizational, require a facilitating environment to be effective. The emphasis on tools for understanding and tools for action brings structure to what can often be emotional and chaotic experience. It is a task-focused, goal-setting approach where recognition of work stress promotes acknowledgement of the need for change. The chapter's emphasis on organizational dynamics and solutions as well as individual action encourages a shared approach to the complex, demanding and interdisciplinary nature of social care practice, and to building on the commitment, courage, compassion and care (SSI 1992a) demonstrated regularly by staff. However, management of the personal experience of work begins with a personal decision to take responsibility for survival and growth, and to join with others in this task, by beginning dialogue, stimulating support systems and initiating change.

The dialogue envisaged throughout this book includes the following.

- An overview – pulling back to analyse practice, the interactions and interrelationships within the system, and to communicate about them, with a view to answering a fundamental question: in which part of the system does the problem reside?
- Personal statements – sharing beliefs, anxieties, values and attitudes about the task, together with outside pressures which seek to influence the direction taken in practice.
- Role negotiation – discussing tasks, difficulties, practice realities and the feelings associated with them. This may involve clarifying the mandate given by the agency and identifying where support may be found for promoting partnership, empowerment and anti-oppressive practice. To remain silent about practice realities and to struggle alone with role conflicts is to collude with the status quo, with the compromises often demanded of practitioners (Preston-Shoot and Agass 1990). What is envisaged here is open communication on how practitioners and users might achieve change.
- Future-oriented questions – dialogue focusing on defining the optimum social care service, and on the means to provide it. Once again the challenge is to avoid merely redoubling efforts, for this will perpetuate the dilemmas and confusions explored in this book. The challenge is to open up the system for change by debating the nature of current provision, understanding users' experiences and illuminating what could be.

Bibliography

Adams, R. (1990). *Self Help, Social Work and Empowerment*. London, Macmillan.

Adams, R. (1993). 'Using the law in social work: a flexible learning initiative?', *Social Work Education*, **12** (special issue), 20–7.

Addison, C. (1982). 'A defence against the public? Aspects of intake in a social services department', *British Journal of Social Work*, **12**(6), 605–18.

Ahmad, A. (1990). *Practice with Care*. London, NISW Race Equality Unit.

Ahmad, B. (ed.) (1990). *Working with the Strengths of Black Families*. London, REU/NISW/LBTC Training for Care.

Ahmad, B. (1991). *Equal Opportunity Training. A Guide for Practice*. London, NISW Race Equality Unit.

Ahmad-Aziz, A., Froggatt, A., Richardson, I., Whittaker, T. and Leung, T. (1992). *Improving Practice with Elders. A Training Manual*. London, Northern Curriculum Development Project, CCETSW.

Allen, I., Hogg, D. and Peace, S. (1993). 'Elderly people – choice, participation and satisfaction', in D. Robbins (ed.) *Community Care. Findings from Department of Health Funded Research, 1988–1992*. London, HMSO.

Allen, P., Thomas, D. and Wakeford, P. (1992). 'Visions for the services', in CCETSW, *Learning Together. Shaping New Services for People with Learning Disabilities*. London, CCETSW.

Arber, S. and Gilbert, N. (1993). 'Men: the forgotten carers', in J. Walmsley, J. Reynolds, P. Shakespeare and R. Woolfe (eds) *Health, Welfare and Practice. Reflecting on Roles and Relationships*. London, Sage/The Open University.

Arnold, P., Bochel, H., Brochurst, S. and Page, D. (1993). 'Accommodation addressed', *Community Care*, 5 August, 18–19.

Arnstein, S. (1969). 'A ladder of citizen participation in the USA', *Journal of the American Institute of Planners*, **35**(4), 216–24.

Atkinson, J. (1991). 'Autonomy and mental health', in P. Barker and S. Baldwin (eds) *Ethical Issues in Mental Health*. London, Chapman and Hall.

Audit Commission (1985). *Managing Social Services for the Elderly More Effectively*. London, HMSO.

Audit Commission (1986). *Making a Reality of Community Care*. London, HMSO.
Audit Commission (1992). *Homeward Bound. A New Course for Community Health*. London, HMSO.
Bacon, R. (1988). 'Counter-transference in a case conference; resistance and rejection in work with abusing families and their children', in G. Pearson, J. Treseder and M. Yelloly (eds) *Social Work and the Legacy of Freud. Psychoanalysis and Its Uses*. London, Macmillan.
Baker, R. (1986). 'The experience of burn-out among social workers: towards an understanding of behavioural reactions', in M. Marshall, M. Preston-Shoot and E. Wincott (eds) *Skills for Social Workers in the 80s*. Birmingham, British Association of Social Workers.
Baldock, J. and Ungerson, C. (1991). '"What d'ya want if you don' want money?" A feminist critique of paid volunteering', in M. Maclean and D. Groves (eds) *Women's Issues in Social Policy*. London, Routledge.
Baldwin, S. (1986). 'Problems with needs – where theory meets practice', *Disability, Handicap and Society*, **1**(2), 139–45.
Baldwin, S. and Parker, G. (1990). 'The Griffith Report on community care', in M. Brenton and C. Ungerson (eds) *Social Policy Review 1988–89*. London, Longman.
Baldwin, S. and Twigg, J. (1991). 'Women and community care. Reflections on a debate', in M. Maclean and D. Groves (eds) *Women's Issues in Social Policy*. London, Routledge.
Balen, R., Brown, K. and Taylor, C. (1993). '"It seems so much is expected of us": practice teachers, the Diploma in Social Work and anti-discriminatory practice', *Social Work Education*, **12**(3), 17–40.
Bamford, T. (1989). 'Discretion and managerialism', in S. Shardlow (ed.) *The Values of Change in Social Work*. London, Tavistock.
Bamford, T. (1990). 'Managing change: buying and providing services', *Social Work Today*, 22 February, 18.
Bano, A., Crosskill, D., Patel, R., Rashman, L. and Shah, R. (1993). *Improving Practice with People with Learning Disabilities*. Leeds, CCETSW Northern Curriculum Development Project.
Barber, J. (1991). *Beyond Casework*. London, Macmillan.
Barclay Report (1982). *Social Workers. Their Role and Tasks*. London, Bedford Square Press.
Barker, I. (1991). *Power Games*. Hove, Pavilion.
Barker, I. and Peck, E. (1987). *Power in Strange Places*. London, Good Practices in Mental Health.
Barnes, C. (1992). 'Institutional discrimination against disabled people and the campaign for anti-discrimination legislation', *Critical Social Policy*, **34**, 12(1), 5–22.
Barnes, M., Bowl, R. and Fisher, M. (1990). *Sectioned: Social Services and the 1983 Mental Health Act*. London, Routledge.
Barton, L. (1993). 'The struggle for citizenship: the case of disabled people', *Disability, Handicap and Society*, **8**(3), 235–48.
BASW (1990). *Community Care: Whose Choice?* Birmingham, British Association of Social Workers.
Baxter, C., Poonia, K., Ward, L. and Nadirshaw, Z. (1990). *Double Discrimination. Issues and Services for People with Learning Difficulties from Black and Ethnic Minority Communities*. London, The Kings Fund Centre.
Bayley, M. (1973). *Mental Handicap and Community Care*. London, Routledge and Kegan Paul.
Bean, P. and Mounser, P. (1993). *Discharged from Mental Hospitals*. London, Macmillan/Mind Publications.
Bebbington, A. and Charnley, H. (1990). 'Community care for the elderly – rhetoric and reality', *British Journal of Social Work*, **20**(5), 409–32.

Bebbington, A. and Davies, B. (1993). 'Efficient targeting of community care: the use of the home help service', *Journal of Social Policy*, **22**(3), 373–91.

Beeforth, M., Coulan, E., Field, V., Hoser, B. and Sayle, L. (eds) (1990). *Whose Service Is It Anyway? Users' Views on Co-ordinating Community Care*. London, Research and Development in Psychiatry.

Bell, L. (1993). 'Home alone', *Community Care* (inside supplement on community care training), 25 February, iv–v.

Benbow, S., Egan, D., Marriott, A., Tregay, K., Walsh, S., Wells, J. and Wood, J. (1990). 'Using the family life cycle with later life families', *Journal of Family Therapy*, **12**, 321–40.

Bennett, P., Evans, R. and Tattersall, A. (1993). 'Stress and coping in social workers. A preliminary investigation', *British Journal of Social Work*, **23**(1), 31–44.

Beresford, P. (1993). 'A programme for change: current issues in user involvement and empowerment', in P. Beresford and T. Harding (eds), *A Challenge to Change. Practical Experiences of Building User Led Services*. London, NISW.

Beresford, P. (1994). 'Blunt talking at the sharp end of welfare', *The Guardian*, 30 March, 13.

Beresford, P. and Croft, S. (1990). 'A sea change', *Community Care*, 4 October, 30–1.

Beresford, P. and Croft, S. (1993). *Citizen Involvement. A Practical Guide for Change*. London, Macmillan.

Bernard, L., Burton, J., Kyne, P. and Simon, J. (1988). 'Groups for older people in residential and day-care: the other groupworkers', *Groupwork*, **1**(2), 115–23.

Biehal, N. and Sainsbury, E. (1991). 'From values to rights in social work. Some issues in practice development and research', *British Journal of Social Work*, **21**(3), 245–57.

Biestek, F. (1957). *The Casework Relationship*. London, Unwin.

Biggs, S. (1990). 'Consumers, case management and inspection: obscuring social deprivation and need?', *Critical Social Policy*, **10**(3), 23–38.

Biggs, S. (1993). 'Hearing their voices', *Community Care* (inside supplement on community care training), 25 February, iii–iv.

Biggs, S. and Weinstein, S. (1991). *Assessment, Care Management and Inspection in Community Care*. London, CCETSW.

Bond, M. (1992). 'Time is on our side', *Social Work Today*, 27 February, 24–6.

Booth, T., Bilson, A. and Fowell, I. (1990). 'Staff attitudes and caring practices in homes for the elderly', *British Journal of Social Work*, **20**(2), 117–31.

Booth, W., Booth, T. and Simons, K. (1988). 'Stepping out: from hostel to independent living', *Practice*, 2(4), 301–10.

Bornat, J. (1993). 'Anthology. Charters', in J. Bornat, C. Pereira, D. Pilgrim and F. Williams (eds) *Community Care. A Reader*. Basingstoke, Macmillan/The Open University.

Borsay, A. (1986). 'Personal trouble or public issue? Towards a model of policy for people with physical and mental disabilities', *Disability, Handicap and Society*, **1**(2), 179–95.

Bould, M. (1990). 'Consultation forums with carers', in L. Winn (ed.) *Power to the People. The Key to Responsive Services in Health and Social Care*. London, The Kings Fund Centre.

Bovaird, T. and Mallinson, I. (1988). 'Setting objectives and measuring achievement in social care', *British Journal of Social Work*, **18**(3), 309–23.

Bowman, G. and Jeffcoat, P. (1990). 'The application of systems ideas in a social services field-work team', *Journal of Family Therapy*, **12**, 243–54.

Boyes, J. (1993). 'Quality in staff development', *Social Work Education*, **12**(2), 5–18.

Bradshaw, J. (1972). 'The concept of social need', *New Society*, **19**(496), 640–3.

Brady, J. (1992). 'Brave new breed', *Community Care* (inside supplement), 27 February, i–ii.

Brandon, D. (1991a). 'The implications of normalisation work for professional skills', in S. Ramon (ed.) *Beyond Community Care. Normalisation and Integration Work.* London, Macmillan.

Brandon, D. (1991b). *Innovation without Change. Consumer Power in Psychiatric Services.* London, Macmillan.

Braye, S. and Preston-Shoot, M. (1992a). *Practising Social Work Law.* London, Macmillan.

Braye, S. and Preston-Shoot, M. (1992b). 'Honourable intentions: partnership and written agreements in welfare legislation', *Journal of Social Welfare and Family Law,* **6**, 511–28.

Braye, S. and Preston-Shoot, M. (1993a). 'Partnership practice: responding to the challenge, realising the potential', *Social Work Education,* **12**(2), 35–53.

Braye, S. and Preston-Shoot, M. (1993b). 'Empowerment and partnership in mental health: towards a different relationship', *Journal of Social Work Practice,* **7**(2), 115–28.

Braye, S. and Preston-Shoot, M. (1994). 'Partners in community care? Rethinking the relationship between the law and social work practice', *Journal of Social Welfare and Family Law,* **2**, 163–83.

Braye, S. and Varley, M. (1992). 'A forgotten dimension? Developing a mental health perspective in social work practice', *Social Work Education,* **11**(2), 41–59.

Brearley, P. (1982). *Risk and Social Work.* London, Routledge, Kegan Paul.

Brindle, D. (1992). 'Life on the edge of an elephant trap', *The Guardian,* 29 April, 25.

Brindle, D. (1993). 'Prejudices dictate care services', *The Guardian,* 29 October, 9.

Brown, A. (1990). 'Groupwork with a difference: the group "mosaic" in residential and day care settings', *Groupwork,* **3**(3), 269–85.

Brown, H. C. (1992). 'Lesbians, the state and social work practice', in M. Langan and L. Day (eds) *Women, Oppression and Social Work: Issues in Anti-Discriminatory Practice.* London, Routledge.

Brown, S. and Griffiths, T. (1993). 'Community mental handicap teams: organisation and operation', in D. Robbins (ed.) *Community Care. Findings from Department of Health Funded Research, 1988–1992.* London, HMSO.

Bulmer, M. (1987). *The Social Basis of Community Care.* London, Allen and Unwin.

Butler, L. (1991). 'Accrediting women's unpaid work and experience', *Adults Learning,* **2**(7), 198–9.

Butt, J., Gorbach, P. and Ahmad, B. (1991). *Equally Fair? A Report on Social Service Departments' Development, Implementation, and Monitoring of Services for the Black and Minority Ethnic Community.* London, REU/NISW.

Byng-Hall, J. (1980). 'Symptom bearer as marital distance regulator: clinical implications?', *Family Process,* **19**, 355–65.

Bynoe, I., Oliver, M. and Barnes, C. (1991). *Equal Rights for Disabled People. The Case for a New Law.* London, Institute for Public Policy Research.

Bywaters, P. (1987). 'The future for social work and nursing', *Social Work Today,* 16 March, 11–13.

Bywaters, P. (1991). 'Case finding and screening for social work in acute general hospitals', *British Journal of Social Work,* **21**(1), 19–39.

Caldock, K. (1993). 'Service histories of elderly people', in D. Robbins (ed.) *Community Care. Findings from Department of Health Funded Research, 1988–1992.* London, HMSO.

Cambridge, P. (1992). 'Case management in community services: organisational responses', *British Journal of Social Work,* **22**(5), 495–517.

Campbell, P. (1990). 'Mental health self advocacy', in L. Winn (ed.) *Power to the People. The Key to Responsive Services in Health and Social Care.* London, The Kings Fund Centre.

Care Sector Consortium (1992). *National Occupational Standards for Care.* London, Care Sector Consortium.

Carl, D. and Jurkovic, G. (1983). 'Agency triangles: problems in agency–family relationships', *Family Process,* **22**, 441–51.

Carr, A. (1989). 'Countertransference reactions to families where child abuse has occurred', *Journal of Family Therapy,* **11**(1), 87–97.

Carson, D. (1988). 'Risk-taking policies', *Journal of Social Welfare Law*, **5**, 328–32.

Casement, P. (1985). *On Learning from the Patient*. London, Tavistock.

CCETSW (1976). *Values in Social Work*. Paper 13. London, CCETSW.

CCETSW (1991a). *Setting the Context for Change: Anti-racist Social Work Education*. Leeds, CCETSW Northern Curriculum Development Project.

CCETSW (1991b). *Rules and Requirements for the Diploma in Social Work*. Paper 30 (second edition). London, CCETSW.

CCETSW (1992a). *Learning Together. Shaping New Services for People with Learning Difficulties*. London, CCETSW.

CCETSW (1992b). *National Vocational Qualifications in Care. Guidance on Approval of Assessment Arrangements*. Paper 29.1. London, CCETSW.

Cecchin, G. (1987). 'Hypothesising, circularity and neutrality revisited: an invitation to curiosity', *Family Process*, **26**(4), 405–13.

Centre for Policy on Ageing (1984). *Home Life: a Code of Practice for Residential Care*. London, CPA.

Centre for Policy on Ageing (1990). *Community Life: a Code of Practice for Community Care*. London, CPA.

Cervi, B. (1993a). 'Complaints persist as SSDs claim success', *Community Care*, 28 October, 2.

Cervi, B. (1993b). 'Report', *Community Care*, 18 March, 1.

Cervi, B. and Marchant, C. (1993). 'Client wins right to choose home', *Community Care*, 8 July, 1.

Challis, D., Chessum, R., Chesterman, J., Luckett, R. and Woods, B. (1988). 'Community care for the frail elderly: an urban experiment', *British Journal of Social Work*, **18** (supplement), 13–42.

Challis, D. and Davies, B. (1986). *Case Management in Community Care*. Aldershot, Gower.

Challis, D. and Davies, B. (1993). 'Case management studies: an overview of the Kent, Gateshead, Darlington and Lewisham findings', in D. Robbins (ed.) *Community Care. Findings from Department of Health Funded Research, 1988–1992*. London, HMSO.

Chamberlin, J. (1988). *On Our Own*. London, Mind.

Cheetham, J. (1989). 'Values in action', in S. Shardlow (ed.) *The Values of Change in Social Work*. London, Tavistock.

Clarke, S. (1993). 'Rough with the smooth', *Community Care*, 9 December, 6–7.

Clode, D. (1992a). 'Best laid plans', *Community Care*, 30 April, 18–20.

Clode, D. (1992b). 'Can we trust the trusts?', *Community Care*, 13 August, 12–13.

Cohen, P. (1992). 'Life in the fast lane', *Social Work Today*, 1 October, 15.

Common, R. and Flynn, N. (1992), *Contracting for Care*. York, Joseph Rowntree Foundation.

Cooper, C. and Marshall, J. (1978). 'Sources of managerial and white collar stress', in C. Cooper and R. Payne (eds) *Stress at Work*. Chichester, Wiley.

Cooper, J. (1990). *The Legal Rights Manual. A Guide for Social Workers and Advice Centres*. Aldershot, Gower.

Coote, A. (ed.) (1992). *The Welfare of Citizens. Developing New Social Rights*. London, Institute for Public Policy Research.

Corden, J. and Preston-Shoot, M. (1987). *Contracts in Social Work*. Aldershot, Gower.

Corney, R. (1993). 'Interprofessional collaboration in mental health care', in D. Robbins (ed.) *Community Care. Findings from Department of Health Funded Research, 1988–1992*. London, HMSO.

Cornwell, N. (1992/3). 'Assessment and accountability in community care', *Critical Social Policy*, **36**, 12(3), 40–52.

Coulshed, V. (1993). 'Adult learning: implications for teaching in social work education', *British Journal of Social Work*, **23**(1), 1–13.

Croft, S. and Beresford, P. (1990). *From Paternalism to Participation. Involving People in Social Services*. London, Open Services Project.

Croft, S. and Beresford, P. (1993). *Getting Involved. A Practical Manual.* London, Open Services Project.

Cummings, T. and Cooper, C. (1979). 'A cybernetic framework for studying occupational stress', *Human Relations*, **32**(5), 395–418.

Dagnan, D. and Drewett, R. (1988). 'Community-based care for people with a mental handicap: a family placement scheme in County Durham', *British Journal of Social Work*, 18(6), 543–75.

Dalley, G. (1988). *Ideologies of Caring: Rethinking Community and Collectivism.* London, Macmillan.

Dalley, G. (1993). 'Professional ideology or organizational tribalism?', in J. Walmsley, J. Reynolds, P. Shakespeare and R. Woolfe (eds) *Health, Welfare and Practice. Reflecting on Roles and Relationships.* London, Sage/The Open University.

Darbyshire, P. (1991). 'Working with people with a mental handicap', in P. Barker and S. Baldwin (eds) *Ethical Issues in Mental Health.* London, Chapman and Hall.

Dare, J., Goldberg, D. and Walinets, R. (1990). 'What is the question you need to answer? How consultation can prevent professional systems immobilizing families', *Journal of Family Therapy*, **12**, 355–69.

Davies, B. (1988). 'Review article: making a reality of community care', *British Journal of Social Work*, **18**, supplement, 173–87.

Davies, B. and Challis, D. (1986). *Matching Resources to Needs in Community Care.* Aldershot, Gower.

Davies, B. and Knapp, M. (1988). 'Introduction: the production of welfare approach: some new PSSRU argument and results', *British Journal of Social Work*, **18** (supplement), 1–11.

Davies, B. and Missiakoulis, S. (1988). 'Heineken and matching processes in the Thanet Community Care Project: an empirical test of their relative importance', *British Journal of Social Work*, **18**, supplement, 55–78.

Davies, M. and Brandon, M. (1988). 'The summer of "88"', *Community Care*, **733**, 16–18.

Davis, K. (1991). 'User participation in Derbyshire', in C. Thompson (ed.) *Changing the Balance. Power and People who Use Services.* London, NCVO.

Day, P. (1987). 'Mind the gap. Normalisation theory and practice', *Practice*, **1**(2), 105–15.

De Board, R. (1978). *The Psychoanalysis of Organisations.* London, Tavistock.

DHSS (1971a). *Hospital Services for the Mentally Ill.* London, HMSO.

DHSS (1971b). *Better Services for the Mentally Handicapped.* London, HMSO.

DHSS (1972). *Services for Mental Illness Related to Old Age.* London, HMSO.

DHSS (1975). *Better Services for the Mentally Ill.* London, HMSO.

DHSS (1981). *Care in the Community. A Consultative Document on Moving Resources for Care in England.* London, DHSS.

DHSS (1983). *Care in the Community.* HC(83)6/LAC(83)5. London, HMSO.

Dimmock, B. and Dungworth, D. (1983). 'Creating manoeuvrability for family/systems therapists in social services departments', *Journal of Family Therapy*, **5**(1), 53–69.

DoH (1988). *Protecting Children. A Guide for Social Workers Undertaking a Comprehensive Assessment.* London, HMSO.

DoH (1989a). *Caring for People: Community Care in the Next Decade and Beyond.* London, HMSO.

DoH (1989b). *The Discharge of Patients from Hospital.* HC(89)5. London, Department of Health.

DoH (1989c). *Homes Are for Living in.* London, HMSO.

DoH (1989d). *The Care of Children. Principles and Practices in Regulations and Guidance.* London, HMSO.

DoH (1990a). *Community Care in the Next Decade and Beyond. Policy Guidance*. London, HMSO.

DoH (1990b). *The Care Programme Approach for People with a Mental Illness Referred to the Specialist Psychiatric Services*. HC(90)23/LAC(90)11. London, Department of Health.

DoH (1990c). *Specific Grant for the Development of Social Care Services for People with a Mental Illness*. HC(90)24/LAC(90)10. London, Department of Health.

DoH (1990d). *Caring for Quality. Guidance on Standards for Residential Homes for Elderly People*. London, HMSO.

DoH (1991a). *Implementing Community Care. Purchaser, Commissioner and Provider Roles*. London, HMSO.

DoH (1991b). *Care Management and Assessment: a Practitioner's Guide*. London, HMSO.

DoH (1991c). *Getting the Message Across. A Guide to Developing and Communicating Policies, Principles and Procedures on Assessment*. London, HMSO.

DoH (1991d). *Purchase of Service. Practice Guidance*. London, HMSO.

DoH (1991e). *Care Management and Assessment. Summary of Practice Guidance*. London, HMSO.

DoH (1991f). *Care Management and Assessment. Managers' Guide*. London, HMSO.

DoH (1991g). *The Right to Complain. Practice Guidance on Complaints Procedures in Social Services Departments*. London, HMSO.

DoH (1991h). *Inspecting for Quality*. London, HMSO.

DoH (1991i). *Working Together. A Guide to Arrangements for Inter-agency Co-operation for the Protection of Children from Abuse*. London, HMSO.

DoH (1991j). *Assessment Systems and Community Care*. London, HMSO.

DoH (1992a). 'Letter from Laming to local authorities', 14 December, Ref. C1/92/34.

DoH (1992b). *Committed to Quality. Quality Assurance in Social Services Departments*. London, HMSO.

DoH (1992c). *Implementing Community Care. Improving Independent Sector Involvement in Community Care Planning*. London, HMSO.

DoH (1993a). *Mental Illness Specific Grant. Second Report on Monitoring Its Use*. London, HMSO.

DoH (1993b). *Training for the Future. Training and Development Guidance to Support the Implementation of the NHS and Community Care Act 1990 and the Full Range of Community Care Reforms*. London, HMSO.

DoH (1993c). *The Health and Social Care of People with HIV Infection and Aids*. London, HMSO.

DoH (1993d). *Code of Practice: Section 118 Mental Health Act 1983*. London, HMSO.

DoH (1993e). 'Letter to local authorities on community care, SSI/RHA monitoring, and priority areas for long-term development', from Herbert Laming and Alan Langlands, Ref: CI(93)35.

DoH (1994). *Report of the Inquiry into the Care and Treatment of Christopher Clunis*. London, HMSO.

Dominelli, L. (1988). *Anti-racist Social Work*. London, Macmillan.

Dominelli, L. and McLeod, E. (1989). *Feminist Social Work*. London, Macmillan.

Douglas, R. and Payne, C. (1988). *Organising for Learning. Staff Development Strategies for Residential and Day Services Work. A Theoretical and Practical Guide*. London, NISW.

Dourado, P. (1991). 'Getting the message across', *Community Care*, 21 March, 22–3.

Doyal, L. (1993). 'Human need and the moral right to optimal community care', in J. Bornat, C. Pereira, D. Pilgrim and F. Williams (eds) *Community Care. A Reader*. Basingstoke, Macmillan/The Open University.

Doyal, L. and Gough, I. (1991). *A Theory of Human Need*. London, Macmillan.

Drake, R. (1992). 'Consumer participation: the voluntary sector and the concept of power', *Disability, Handicap and Society*, **7**(3), 267–78.

Dugmore, J. (1991). 'Language lessons', *Community Care*, 7 February, 24–6.

Dungworth, D. (1988). 'Context and the construction of family therapy practice', in E. Street and W. Dryden (eds) *Family Therapy in Britain*. Milton Keynes, Open University Press.

Dungworth, D. and Reimers, S. (1984). 'Family therapy in social services departments', in A. Treacher and J. Carpenter (eds) *Using Family Therapy*. Oxford, Basil Blackwell.

Dutt, R. (ed.) (1990). *Black Community and Community Care*. London, REU/NISW.

Dyer, C. (1993). 'Challenging state in court "a lottery"', *The Guardian*, 21 June, 4.

Ellis, K. (1993). *Squaring the Circle. User and Carer Participation in Needs Assessment*. York, Joseph Rowntree Foundation.

England, H. (1986). *Social Work as Art*. London, Allen and Unwin.

Erlichman, J. (1994). 'New charity helps 50 whistleblowers', *The Guardian*, 17 January, 4.

Fairbairn, G. (1987). 'Responsibility, respect for persons and psychological change', in S. Fairbairn and G. Fairbairn (eds) *Psychology, Ethics and Change*. London, RKP.

Fairbairn, S. and Fairbairn, G. (eds) (1987). *Psychology, Ethics and Change*. London, Routledge and Kegan Paul.

Fennell, P. (1990). 'Inscribing paternalism in the law: consent to treatment and mental disorder', *Journal of Law and Society*, **17**(1), 29–51.

Fernando, S. (1991). *Mental Health, Race and Culture*. London, Macmillan.

Finch, J. (1984). 'Community care: developing non-sexist alternatives', *Critical Social Policy*, **9**, 6–18.

Finkelstein, V. (1991). 'Disability. An administrative challenge', in M. Oliver (ed.) *Social Work. Disabled People and Disabling Environments*. London, Jessica Kingsley.

Finkelstein, V. (1993a). 'From curing or caring to defining disabled people', in J. Walmsley, J. Reynolds, P. Shakespeare and R. Woolfe (eds) *Health, Welfare and Practice. Reflecting on Roles and Relationships*. London, Sage/The Open University.

Finkelstein, V. (1993b). 'The commonality of disability', in J. Swain, V. Finkelstein, S. French and M. Oliver (eds) *Disabling Barriers – Enabling Environments*. Milton Keynes, Open University/Sage.

Fisher, M. (1990a). 'Defining the practice context of care management', *Social Work and Social Sciences Review*, **2**, 204–30.

Fisher, M. (1990b). 'Care management and social work: clients with dementia', *Practice*, **4**(4), 229–41.

Fisher, M., Newton, C. and Sainsbury, E. (1984). *Mental Health Social Work Observed*. London, George Allen & Unwin.

Flynn, N. and Hurley, D. (1993a). 'The big deal. Purchasing dilemmas', *Community Care*, 28 October, 19.

Flynn, N. and Hurley, D. (1993b). 'Purchasing dilemma 4', *Community Care*, 18 November, 21.

Fox Harding, L. (1991). *Perspectives in Child Care Policy*. London, Longman.

Francis, J. (1992). 'Crisis in the grey area', *Community Care*, 11 June, 26.

Francis, J. (1993). 'Pressure group', *Community Care*, 24 June, 14–15.

Freeden, M. (1991). *Rights*. Buckingham, Open University Press.

French, J. and Raven, (1959). 'The bases of social power', in D. Cartwright (ed.) *Studies in Social Power*. Ann Arbor, University of Michigan Press.

French, S. (1993). 'Disability, impairment or something in between?', in J. Swain, V. Finkelstein, S. French and M. Oliver (eds) *Disabling Barriers – Enabling Environments*. Milton Keynes, Open University/Sage.

Frosh, S. (1987). *The Politics of Psychoanalysis*. London, Macmillan.

Furniss, T. (1983). 'Mutual influence and interlocking professional–family process in the treatment of child sexual abuse and incest', *Child Abuse and Neglect*, **7**, 207–23.

Galligan, D. (1992). 'Procedural rights in social welfare', in A. Coote (ed.) *The Welfare of Citizens. Developing New Social Rights*. London, Rivers Oram Press/IPPR.

Gardener, D. (1988). 'A sharing approach to the management of stress', *Social Work Today*, **20**(7), 18–19.

George, M. (1993). 'Legal storm brewing', *Community Care*, 29 April, 18–19.

Gibbs, I. and Sinclair, I. (1992). 'Consistency: a pre-requisite for inspecting old people's homes?', *British Journal of Social Work*, **22**(5), 535–50.

Gibson, F., McGrath, A. and Reid, N. (1989). 'Occupational stress in social work', *British Journal of Social Work*, **19**(1), 1–18.

Goldberg, D. and Huxley, P. (1992). *Common Mental Disorders. A Bio-social Model*. London, Routledge.

Gomm, R. (1993). 'Issues of power in health and welfare', in J. Walmsley, J. Reynolds, P. Shakespeare and R. Woolfe (eds) *Health, Welfare and Practice. Reflecting on Roles and Relationships*. London, Sage/The Open University.

Goodwin, S. (1990). *Community Care and the Future of Mental Health Service Provision*. Aldershot, Avebury.

Gorman, J. (1992). *Out of the Shadows. Mind Campaigns for Women's Mental Health*. London, Mind.

GPMH and Camden Consortium (1988). *Treated Well? A Code of Practice for Psychiatric Hospitals*. London, Good Practices in Mental Health.

Graham, H. (1993). 'Feminist perspectives on caring', in J. Bornat, C. Pereira, D. Pilgrim and F. Williams (eds) *Community Care. A Reader*. Basingstoke, Macmillan/The Open University.

Grandison, K. (1992). 'Health warning', *Social Work Today*, 22 October, 24.

Griffiths, R. (1988). *Community Care: Agenda for Action*. London, HMSO.

Grimwood, C. and Popplestone, R. (1993). *Women, Management and Care*. London, Macmillan.

Gunaratnam, Y. (1993). 'Breaking the silence: Asian carers in Britain', in J. Bornat, C. Pereira, D. Pilgrim and F. Williams (eds) *Community Care. A Reader*. Basingstoke, Macmillan/The Open University.

Gunn, M. (1991). *Sex and the Law*, 3rd edn. London, Family Planning Association.

Hambleton, R. and Hoggett, P. (1990). *Beyond Excellence: Quality Local Government in the 1990's*. Working Paper 85. Bristol, SAUS.

Handy, C. (1985). *Understanding Organisations*. Harmondsworth, Penguin.

Hanmer, J. and Statham, D. (1988). *Women and Social Work. Towards a Woman-centred Practice*. London, Macmillan.

Hardy, B., Wistow, G., Turrell, A. and Webb, A. (1993) 'Collaboration and cost effectiveness', in D. Robbins (ed.) *Community Care. Findings from Department of Health Funded Research, 1988–1992*. London, HMSO.

Harris, N. (1987). 'Defensive social work', *British Journal of Social Work*, **17**(1), 61–9.

Harris, V. (1991). 'Values of social work in the context of British society in conflict with anti-racism', in CCETSW, *Setting the Context for Change: Anti-racist Social Work Education*. Leeds, CCETSW Northern Curriculum Development Project.

Harvey, M. and Tisdall, C. (1992). *Vocational Qualifications in Care*. Birmingham, Pepar Publications.

Hatfield, B., Huxley, P. and Mohamad, H. (1992/3). 'The support networks of people with severe, long-term mental health problems', *Practice*, **6**(1), 25–40.

Hearn, J. and Morgan, D. (eds) (1990). *Men, Masculinities and Social Theory*. London, Unwin Hyman.

Henderson, P. and Armstrong, S. (1993). 'Community development and community care', in J. Bornat, C. Pereira, D. Pilgrim and F. Williams (eds) *Community Care. A Reader*. Basingstoke, Macmillan/The Open University.

Henwood, M. (1993). 'Smart thinking', *Social Work Today*, 14 January, 18.

Higgins, R. (1992). 'Room to consume', *Social Work Today*, 26 March, 14–15.

Hogman, G. (1992). *Window Dressing. The Care Programme Approach and the Mental Illness Specific Grant. April 1991–April 1992. The First Year*. London, National Schizophrenia Fellowship.

Hollis, F. (1970). 'The psychosocial approach to the practice of casework', in R. Roberts and R. Nee (eds) *Theories of Social Casework*. Chicago, University of Chicago Press.

Horne, M. (1987). *Values in Social Work*. Aldershot, Wildwood House.

House of Commons Social Services Committee (1985). *Community Care*. HCP 13–1, Session 84–85. London, HMSO.

Howe, D. (1979). 'Agency function and social work principles', *British Journal of Social Work*, **9**(1), 29–47.

Hudson, A. with Ayensu, L., Oadley, C. and Patocchi, M. (1993). 'Practising feminist approaches', in C. Hanvey and T. Philpot (eds) *Practising Social Work*. London, Routledge.

Hudson, B. (1990). 'Social policy and the New Right – the strange case of the Community Care White Paper', *Local Government Studies*, November/December, 15–34.

Hudson, B. (1991). 'Quality time', *Health Service Journal*, 12 September, 22–3.

Hughes, B. and Mtezuka, M. (1992). 'Social work and older women: where have older women gone?', in M. Langan and L. Day (eds) *Women, Oppression and Social Work: Issues in Anti-Discriminatory Practice*. London, Routledge.

Hugman, R. (1989). 'Rehabilitation and community care in mental health (1). Some implications for practice', *Practice*, **3**(2), 119–35.

Hugman, R. (1991). *Power in Caring Professions*. London, Macmillan.

Humphries, B. (1993). 'Are you or have you ever been. . .?', *Social Work Education*, **12**(3), 6–8.

Humphries, R. (1992). 'Champions of change', *Community Care*, 29 October, 24–5.

Husband, C. (1991). ' "Race", conflictual politics and anti-racist social work: lessons from the past for action in the 1990's', in CCETSW, *Setting the Context for Change: Anti-racist Social Work Education*. Leeds, CCETSW Northern Curriculum Development Project.

Hutchinson, M. and McAusland, T. (1993) 'Learning about user involvement', in NHSTD, *Training and User Involvement in Mental Health Services*. London, National Health Service Training Directorate with Survivors Speak Out, Mindlink and National Advocacy Network.

Huxley, P. (1990). 'The relationship between health care and social care in the provision of community care for mentally ill people', a summary paper for the North West and Merseyside Regions Conference, 26 June.

Huxley, P. (1993). 'Case management and care management in community care', *British Journal of Social Work*, **23**(4), 365–81.

Huxley, P., Mohamad, H., Korer, J., Jacob, C., Raval, H. and Anthony, P. (1993). 'The prevalence and outcome of minor psychiatric disorders in social work clients', in D. Robbins (ed.) *Community Care. Findings from Department of Health Funded Research, 1988–1992*. London, HMSO.

Illich, I. (1975). *Medical Nemesis. The Expropriation of Health*. London, Calder and Boyars.

Inner London Probation Service (undated). *Working with Difference. A Positive and Practical Guide to Anti-discriminatory Practice Teaching*. London, ILPS with Greater London Probation Pre-Service Training Committee and Tuklo Associates.

Isaac, B. (1991). 'Negotiation in partnership work', in Family Rights Group, *The Children Act 1989: Working in Partnership with Parents. Reader*. London, HMSO.

Ivory, M. (1993). 'Report', *Community Care*, 1 April, 1.

Jadeja, S. and Singh, J. (1993). 'Life in a cold climate', *Community Care*, 22 April, 12–13.

Janis, I. (1972). *Victims of Groupthink: a Psychological Study of Foreign Policy Decisions and Fiascos*. Boston, Houghton Mifflin.

Janner, G. (1990). 'More than just keeping up the quotas', *Social Work Today*, **21**(18), 23.

Jaques, E. (1955). 'Social systems as defence against persecutory and depressive anxiety', in M. Klein, P. Heimann and R. Money-Kyrle (eds) *New Directions in Psychoanalysis*. London, Tavistock.

Johnstone, L. (1989). *Users and Abusers of Psychiatry*. London, Routledge.

Jones, A., Phillips, M. and Maynard, C. (1992). *A Home from Home. The Experience of Black Residential Projects as a Focus of Good Practice*. London, REU/NISW.

Jones, C. (1993). 'The right and anti-racist social work education', *Social Work Education*, **12**(3), 9–16.

Jones, C. and Novak, T. (1993). 'Social work today', *British Journal of Social Work*, **23**(3), 195–212.

Jones, F., Fletcher, B. and Ibbetson, K. (1991). 'Stressors and strains amongst social workers: demands, supports, constraints, and psychological health', *British Journal of Social Work*, **21**(5), 443–69.

Jordan, B. (1991). 'Competencies and values', *Social Work Education*, **10**(1), 5–11.

Joseph Rowntree Foundation (1992). *Using Training to Improve Services. Social Care Research Findings No. 20*. York, Joseph Rowntree Foundation.

Keep, J. (1992). 'Stand and deliver', *Community Care*, 27 August, 12–13.

Keith, L. (1990). 'Caring partnership', *Community Care* (inside supplement), 22 February, v–vi.

Kelly, D. (1993). 'Suspicious minds', *Community Care*, 10 June, 6.

Kelly, D., Payne, C. and Warwick, J. (1990). *Making National Vocational Qualifications Work for Social Care*. London, NISW/SCA.

Kemsall, H. (1993). 'Assessing competence: scientific process or subjective inference? Do we really see it?', *Social Work Education*, **12**(1), 36–45.

King, J. (1991). 'Taking the strain', *Community Care*, 24 October, 16–18.

Kings Fund (1983). *An Ordinary Life*. London, The Kings Fund Centre.

Kitwood, T. and Bredin, K. (1992). *Person to Person. A Guide to the Care of Those with Failing Mental Powers*. Loughton, Gale Centre Publications.

Kitzinger, J., Green, J. and Coupland, V. (1993). 'Labour relations: midwives and doctors on the labour ward', in J. Walmsley, J. Reynolds, P. Shakespeare, and R. Woolfe (eds) *Health, Welfare and Practice. Reflecting on Roles and Relationships*. London, Sage/The Open University.

Knapp, M. (1993). 'Care in the community demonstration programme', in D. Robbins (ed.) *Community Care. Findings from Department of Health Funded Research, 1988–1992*. London, HMSO.

Knapp, M., Cambridge, P., Thomason, C., Beecham, J., Allen, C. and Darton, R. (1992). *Care in the Community: Challenge and Demonstration*. Aldershot, PSSRU/Ashgate.

Lambert, D. (1993). *Letter to London Authorities*. London, SSI/DoH.

Land, H. (1991). 'Time to care', in M. Maclean and D. Groves (eds) *Women's Issues in Social Policy*. London, Routledge.

Langan, M. (1990). 'Community care in the 1990s: the community care White Paper "Caring for People"', *Critical Social Policy*, **10**(2), 58–70.

Langan, M. (1992) 'Introduction: women and social work in the 1990s', in M. Langan and L. Day (eds) *Women, Oppression and Social Work: Issues in Anti-Discriminatory Practice*. London, Routledge.

Law Commission (1993). *Mentally Incapacitated Adults and Decision-making. A New Jurisdiction*. Consultation Paper No. 128. London, HMSO.

Lawler, J. (1994). 'A competence based approach to management education in social work: a discussion of the approach and its relevance', *Social Work Education*, **13**(1), 60–82.

Lawson, M. (1991). 'A recipient's view', in S. Ramon (ed.) *Beyond Community Care. Normalisation and Integration Work*. London, Macmillan.

Lawton, D. and Parker, G. (1993). 'Analysis of 1985 General Household Survey data on informal care', in D. Robbins (ed.) *Community Care. Findings from Department of Health Funded Research, 1988–1992*. London, HMSO.

LBTC (1992). *Purchase of Service Training Guidelines*. London, London Borough Training Consortium, Training for Care/DoH.

Leedham, I. and Wistow, G. (1993). 'Just what the doctor ordered', *Community Care*, 7 January, 22–3.

Levick, P. (1992). 'The Janus face of community care legislation: an opportunity for radical possibilities?', *Critical Social Policy*, **12**(1), 75–92.

Lewis, A. (1991). 'Public participation in decision-making', in S. Ramon (ed.) *Beyond Community Care. Normalisation and Integration Work*. London, Macmillan.

Lewis, J. (1993). 'Developing the mixed economy of care: emerging issues for voluntary organisations', *Journal of Social Policy*, **22**(2), 173–92.

Lindow, V. (1992). 'Just lip service?', *Nursing Times*, 2 December, 63.

Llewelyn, S. (1987). 'Ethical issues in psychotherapy for women', in S. Fairbairn and G. Fairbairn (eds) *Psychology, Ethics and Change*. London, Routledge and Kegan Paul.

Lloyd, M. (1992). 'Does she boil eggs? Towards a feminist model of disability', *Disability, Handicap and Society*, **7**(2), 207–22.

Loden, M. (1985). *Feminine Leadership. How to Succeed in Business Without Being One of the Boys*. London, Times Books.

Lonsdale, S. (1990). *Women and Disability*. London, Macmillan.

Lukes, S. (1974). *Power: a Radical View*. London, Macmillan.

McCalman, J. (1990). *The Forgotten People: Carers in Three Minority Ethnic Communities in Southwark*. London, The Kings Fund Centre.

McCarthy, M. and Thompson, D. (1991). 'The politics of sex education', *Community Care*, 21 November, 15–17.

McDonald, J. (1992/3). Quotation from 'From anger to action', printed in *Openmind*, December/January, 11.

Macdonald, S. (1991). *All Equal under the Act?* London, REU/NISW.

McGrath, M. (1993). 'Policy implementation studies – the all-Wales mental handicap strategy', in D. Robbins (ed.) *Community Care. Findings from Department of Health Funded Research, 1988–1992*. London, HMSO.

McNay, M. (1992). 'Work and power relations: towards a framework for an integrated practice', in M. Langan and L. Day (eds) *Women, Oppression and Social Work: Issues in Anti-Discriminatory Practice*. London, Routledge.

Makin, P., Cooper, C. and Cox, C. (1989). *Managing People at Work*. London, Routledge.

Malan, D. (1979). *Individual Psychotherapy and the Science of Psychodynamics*. London, Butterworths.

Mama, A. (1993). 'Violence against black women; gender, race and state responses', in J. Walmsley, J. Reynolds, P. Shakespeare and R. Woolfe (eds) *Health, Welfare and Practice. Reflecting on Roles and Relationships*. London, Sage/The Open University.

Mann, A., Blanchard, M. and Waterreus, A. (1993). 'Community psychiatric nurse management of the elderly depressed in the community – interim report', in D. Robbins (ed.) *Community Care. Findings from Department of Health Funded Research, 1988–1992*. London, HMSO.

Mansell, J. and Beasley, F. (1993). 'Small staffed houses for people with a severe learning disability and challenging behaviour', *British Journal of Social Work*, **23**(4), 329–44.

Marchant, C. (1993). 'Crock of fool's gold?', *Community Care*, 1 April, 14–16.

Marsh, P. and Fisher, M. (1992). *Good Intentions: Developing Partnership in Social Services*. York, Joseph Rowntree Foundation.

Mawhinney, B. (1993). 'Check against delivery', Closing address to the Social Services Conference, 29 October, Solihull.

Mayer, J. and Timms, N. (1970). *The Client Speaks*. London, RKP.

Meade, K. and Carter, T. (1990). 'Empowering older users: some starting points', in L. Winn (ed.) *Power to the People. The Key to Responsive Services in Health and Social Care*. London, The Kings Fund Centre.

Menzies, I. (1970). *The Functioning of Social Systems as a Defence Against Anxiety*. London, Tavistock.

Mihill, C. (1991). 'NHS anti-racism policies "failing"', *The Guardian*, 21 January, 7.

Miller, C. (1991). 'Split vision', *Social Work Today*, 19 September, 24–5.

Milroy, A. and Hennelley, R. (1989). 'Changing our professional ways', in A. Brackx and C. Grimshaw (eds) *Mental Health Care in Crisis*. London, Pluto Press.

Mind (1983). *Common Concern – Manifesto for a New Mental Health Service*. London, Mind.

Mind (1992). *The Mind Guide to Advocacy*. London, Mind.

Mirza, K. (1991). 'Community care for the black community – waiting for guidance', in CCETSW, *One Small Step Towards Racial Justice*. London, CCETSW.

Mitchell, D. (1993). 'Slow off the mark', *Community Care*, 11 March, 22–3.

Moonie, N. and Newlyn, B. (1990). 'Competent care depends on competent training', *Social Work Education*, **9**(3), 35–43.

Morris, J. (1991). *Pride against Prejudice. Transforming Attitudes to Disability*. London, Women's Press.

Morris, J. (1991/2). '"Us" and "them"? Feminist research, community care and disability', *Critical Social Policy*, **33**, 11(3), 22–39.

Morris, J. (1993a). 'Key task 1. Criteria motives', *Community Care*, 14 January, 17.

Morris, J. (1993b). 'Achievable goals', *Community Care*, 18 February. 22–3.

Morris, J. (1993c). 'Gender and disability', in J. Swain, V. Finkelstein, S. French and M. Oliver (eds) *Disabling Barriers – Enabling Environments*. London, Sage/The Open University.

Morris, J. (1993d). *Community Care or Independent Living?* York, Joseph Rowntree Foundation.

Mullender, A. (1992/3). 'Disabled people find a voice: will it be heard in the move towards community care?', *Practice*, **6**(1), 5–15.

Mullender, A. and Ward, D. (1991). *Self-Directed Groupwork – Users Take Action for Empowerment*. London, Whiting and Birch.

Murgatroyd, S. (1992). 'Stress at work: a workshop', in T. Hobbs (ed.) *Experiential Training*. London, Routledge.

Murrell, J. (1993). 'Judgement of professional competence: bags of bias', *Social Work Education*, **12** (special issue), 5–19.

Naik, D. (1991). 'An examination of social work education within an anti-racist framework', in CCETSW, *Setting the Context for Change: Anti-racist Social Work Education*. Leeds, CCETSW Northern Curriculum Development Project.

Naik, D. (1993). 'Towards an anti-racist curriculum in social work training', in J. Walmsley, J. Reynolds, P. Shakespeare and R. Woolfe (eds) *Health, Welfare and Practice. Reflecting on Roles and Relationships*. London, Sage/The Open University.

NAREA (undated). *Black Community Care Charter*. Birmingham, National Association of Race Equality Advisers.

NCC (1993). *Getting Heard and Getting Things Changed*. London, National Consumer Council.

NCVS (1989). *A Working Definition of Oppression*. Nottingham, Nottingham Council for Voluntary Service.

Neill, J. (1982). 'Some variations in policy and procedure relating to Part 3 applications in the GLC area', *British Journal of Social Work*, **12**(3), 229–45.

Nelken, D. (1987). 'The use of contracts as a social work technique', *Current Legal Problems*, **40**, 207–32.

Nelken, D. (1989). 'Discipline and punish: some notes on the margin', *The Howard Journal*, **28**(4), 245–54.

Newman, T. (1993). 'Keeping in step', *Community Care* (inside supplement), 28 October, 4–5.

Newton, C. and Marsh, P. (1993). *Training in Partnership. Translating Intentions into Practice in Social Services.* York, Joseph Rowntree Foundation.

NHS Management Executive (1993). *Nursing in Primary Health Care. New World, New Opportunities.* London, NHSME.

NHSTD (1993). *Training and User Involvement in Mental Health Services.* London, National Health Service Training Directorate in collaboration with Survivors Speak Out, Mindlink and the National Advocacy Network.

NISW/NEC (1993). *How to Manage Your Training.* Cambridge, National Institute for Social Work/National Extension College.

Norman, A. (1980). *Rights and Risk. A Discussion Document on Civil Liberty in Old Age.* London, Centre for Policy on Ageing.

North, C., Ritchie, J. and Ward, K. (1993). *Factors Influencing the Implementation of the Care Programme Approach.* London, HMSO.

NUPE (1993). *Bringing It All Home.* London, NUPE.

O'Brian, C. and Bruggen, P. (1985). 'Our personal and professional lives: learning positive connotation and circular questioning', *Family Process*, **24**, 311–22.

O'Brien, J. (1986). 'A guide to personal futures planning', in G. Bellamy and B. Wilcox (eds) *The Activities Catalog: a Community Programming Guide for Youth and Adults with Severe Disabilities.* Baltimore, Paul H. Brookes Publishing Company.

O'Brien, J. (1989). *Nottingham Patients Council Support Group Information Pack.* Nottingham, NPCSG.

Oliver, M. (1991/2). 'Review of Naomi Connelly (1990), Raising Voices: Social Services Departments and People with Disabilities. Policy Studies Institute', *Critical Social Policy*, **33**, 115–16.

Oliver, M. and Barnes, C. (1993). 'Discrimination, disability and welfare: from needs to rights', in J. Swain, V. Finkelstein, S. French and M. Oliver (eds) *Disabling Barriers – Enabling Environments.* Milton Keynes, Open University/Sage.

Onyett, S. (1992). *Case Management in Mental Health.* London, Chapman and Hall.

Orme, J. and Glastonbury, B. (1993). *Care Management.* London, Macmillan.

Ormiston, H. and Haggard, L. (1993). 'A long road ahead', *Community Care*, 17 June, 16–17.

OSDC (1991). *Anti-racist Ways of Working in Training.* Sheffield, Organisation and Social Development Consultants.

O'Sullivan, T. (1990). 'Responding to people with dementia', *Practice*, **4**(1), 5–15.

Øvretveit, J. (1986). *Organisation of Multidisciplinary Community Teams.* Uxbridge, Brunel University Institute of Organisation and Social Studies.

Parker, G. (1993). 'A four-way stretch? The politics of disability and caring', in J. Swain, V. Finkelstein, S. French and M. Oliver (eds) *Disabling Barriers – Enabling Environments.* Milton Keynes, Open University/Sage.

Parsloe, P. (1993). 'Making a bid for fair play', *Community Care*, 5 August, 16–17.

Payne, C. and Scott, T. (1982). *Developing Supervision of Teams in Field and Residential Social Work.* Paper 12. London, NISW.

Payne, M. (1986). *Social Care in the Community.* London, Macmillan.

Payne, M. (1987). 'Residential care with mentally ill people', *Practice*, **1**(3), 213–24.

Payne, M. (1989). 'Open records and shared decisions with clients', in S. Shardlow (ed.) *The Values of Change in Social Work*. London, Tavistock.

Payne, R. and Firth-Cozens, J. (1987). *Stress in Health Professionals*. Chichester, Wiley.

Pelikan, C. (1991). 'A marriage of convenience', *Community Care*, 19 September, 17–19.

Penhale, B. (1993). 'The abuse of elderly people: considerations for practice, *British Journal of Social Work*, **23**(2), 95–112.

Pfeffer, N. and Coote, A. (1991). *Is Quality Good For You? A Critical Review of Quality Assurance in Welfare Services*. London, Institute for Public Policy Research.

Phillipson, J. (1992). *Practising Equality. Women, Men and Social Work*. London, CCETSW.

Pines, A. and Maslach, C. (1980). 'Combating staff burnout in a day care setting', *Child Care Quarterly*, **9**, 5–16.

Plumb, A. (1987). 'That word consumer', *Rochdale and District Mind Newsletter*, 4.

Plumb, A. (1991). 'The challenge of self-advocacy', unpublished paper subsequently amended and published (Plumb, 1993).

Plumb, A. (1993). 'The challenge of self-advocacy', *Feminism and Psychology*, **3**(2), 169–87.

Pottage, D. and Evans, M. (1992). *Workbased Stress: Prescription Is Not the Cure*. London, NISW.

Pottle, S. (1984). 'Developing a network-orientated service for elderly people and their carers', in A. Treacher and J. Carpenter (eds) *Using Family Therapy*. Oxford, Basil Blackwell.

Preston-Shoot, M. (1987). *Effective Groupwork*. London, Macmillan.

Preston-Shoot, M. (1991). 'A model and method for staff and team appraisal', in M. Marshall, M. Preston-Shoot and E. Wincott (eds) *Effective Management*. Birmingham, British Association of Social Workers.

Preston-Shoot, M. (1992). 'On empowerment, partnership, and authority in groupwork practice: a training contribution', *Groupwork*, **5**(2), 5–30.

Preston-Shoot, M. (1994). 'Written agreements: a contractual approach to social work', in C. Hanvey and T. Philpot (eds) *Practising Social Work*. London, Routledge.

Preston-Shoot, M. and Agass, D. (1990). *Making Sense of Social Work: Psychodynamics, Systems and Practice*. London, Macmillan.

Preston-Shoot, M. and Braye, S. (1991). 'Managing the personal experience of work', *Practice*, **5**(1), 13–33.

Prior, L. (1993). *The Social Organisation of Mental Illness*. London, Sage.

Prodgers, A. (1979). 'Defences against stress in intake work', *Social Work Today*, **11**(2), 12–14.

Pugh, G. and De'Ath, E. (1989). *Working towards Partnership in the Early Years*. London, National Children's Bureau.

Purtilo, R. (1993). 'Meaningful distances', in J. Walmsley, J. Reynolds, P. Shakespeare and R. Woolfe (eds) *Health, Welfare and Practice. Reflecting on Roles and Relationships*. London, Sage.

Ramon, S. (1988). 'Skills for normalisation work', *Practice*, **2**(2), 139–49.

Ramon, S. (1991a). 'Preface', in S. Ramon (ed.) *Beyond Community Care. Normalisation and Integration Work*. London, Macmillan.

Ramon, S. (1991b). 'Principles and conceptual knowledge', in S. Ramon (ed.) *Beyond Community Care. Normalisation and Integration Work*. London, Macmillan.

Ramon, S. (1992). 'Working together', *Openmind*, August/September, 28.

Raynes, N. (1993). 'An inspector calls', *Community Care*, 18 March, 26–7.

Read, J. and Wallcraft, J. (1992). *Guidelines for Empowering Users of Mental Health Services*. London, Mind/COHSE.

Reder, P. and Kraemer, S. (1980). 'Dynamic aspects of professional collaboration in child guidance referral', *Journal of Adolescence*, **3**, 165–73.

Rees, S. (1991). *Achieving Power. Practice and Policy in Social Welfare*. North Sydney, Allen and Unwin.

Renshaw, J. (1988). 'Care in the community: individual care planning and case management', *British Journal of Social Work*, **18** (supplement), 79–105.

REU (1989). *Interpreting in Action*. A report of the conference 'Language, Race and Power' held in Newcastle upon Tyne, 11 May. London, Race Equality Unit.

REU (1990). *Black Women in Social Work*. London, NISW/Race Equality Unit.

Reynolds, J. (1993). 'Feminist theory and strategy in social work', in J. Walmsley, J. Reynolds, P. Shakespeare and R. Woolfe (eds) *Health, Welfare and Practice. Reflecting on Roles and Relationships*. London, Sage/The Open University.

Riches, P. (1993). 'Key task 7. Training', *Community Care*, 11 March, 17.

Riches, P. and Whitfield, J. (1992). 'Starting the final lap', *Community Care*, 10 December, 14–16.

Rickford, F. (1993). 'Diamond rings and bathtime', *Community Care*, 21 January, 15–17.

Risdale, L. (1993). *Skill Mix in Primary Care: a Review of Research and Policy in the Past and Present, with Suggestions for the Future*. The Centre for the Advancement of Interprofessional Education Occasional Paper, No. 1. London, CAIPE.

Robbins, D. (ed.) (1993). *Community Care. Findings from Department of Health Funded Research, 1988–1992*. London, HMSO.

Rogers, A., Lacey, R. and Pilgrim, D. (1993). *Experiencing Psychiatry*. London, Macmillan.

Rogers, J. (1990). *Caring for People*. Milton Keynes, Open University Press.

Rojek, C., Peacock, G. and Collins, S. (1988). *Social Work and Received Ideas*. London, Routledge.

Ryan, J. and Thomas, F. (1993). 'Concepts of normalisation', in J. Bornat, C. Pereira, D. Pilgrim and F. Williams (eds) *Community Care. A Reader*. Basingstoke, Macmillan/The Open University.

Sainsbury, E. (1989). 'Participation and paternalism', in S. Shardlow (ed.) *The Values of Change in Social Work*. London, Tavistock.

Sapey, B. and Hewitt, N. (1991). 'The changing context of social work practice', in M. Oliver (ed.) *Social Work, Disabled People and Disabling Environments*. London, Jessica Kingsley.

Sashidharan, S. (1989). 'Schizophrenic – or just black?', *Community Care*, 5 October, 14–15.

Schneider, J. (1993). 'Care programming in mental health: assimilation and adaptation', *British Journal of Social Work*, **23**(4), 383–403.

Schneidman, E. (1985). *Definition of Suicide*. Chichester, Wiley.

Schön, D. (1993). *The Reflective Practitioner*. New York, Basic Books.

Secker, J. (1993). *From Theory to Practice in Social Work*. Aldershot, Avebury.

Seebohm Report (1968). *Report of the Committee on Local Authority and Allied Personal Social Services*. London, HMSO.

Segal, J. (1991). 'The professional perspective', in S. Ramon (ed.) *Beyond Community Care. Normalisation and Integration Work*. London, Macmillan.

Selvini Palazzoli, M., Boscolo, L., Cecchin, G. and Prata, G. (1978). *Paradox and Counterparadox*. New York, Jason Aronson.

Selvini Palazzoli, M., Boscolo, L., Cecchin, G. and Prata, G. (1980). 'The problem of the referring person', *Journal of Marital and Family Therapy*, **6**, 3–9.

Shakespeare, J. (1993). 'Disabled people's self-organisation: a new social movement', *Disability, Handicap and Society*, **8**(3), 249–64.

Shardlow, S. (ed.) (1989). *The Values of Change in Social Work*. London, Tavistock.

Sinclair, I., Stanforth, L. and O'Connor, P. (1988). 'Factors predicting admission of elderly people to local authority residential care', *British Journal of Social Work*, **18**(3), 251–68.

Sivanandan, A. (1991). 'Black struggles against racism', in CCETSW, *Setting the Context for Change: Anti-racist Social Work Education*. Leeds, CCETSW Northern Curriculum Development Project.

Smale, G. (1983). 'Can we afford not to develop social work practice?', *British Journal of Social Work*, **13**(3), 251–64.

Smale, G. and Tuson, G. with Biehal, N. and Marsh, P. (1993). *Empowerment, Assessment, Care Management and the Skilled Worker*. London, NISW/HMSO.

Smith, G. and Harris, R. (1972). 'Ideologies of need and the organisation of social work departments', *British Journal of Social Work*, **2**(1), 27–45.

Smockum, F. (1991). 'Putting women in their place', *The Guardian*, 3 December, 33.

Social Care Association (1988). *Code of Practice for Social Care*. Surbiton, SCA.

Sone, K. (1992). 'Just close your eyes and blow?', *Community Care*, 6 August, 14–15.

Sone, K. (1993). 'Black lives, white perspectives', *Community Care*, 25 March, 14–15.

Spastics Society (1991). *What the Papers Say and Don't Say about Disability*. London, The Spastics Society.

SSI (1989). *Doing It Better Together*. London, DoH.

SSI (1990a). *Training for Community Care. A Strategy*. London, SSI/CCETSW.

SSI (1990b). *Developing Services for Young People with Disabilities*. London, DoH.

SSI (1991a). *Assessment Systems and Community Care*. London, HMSO.

SSI (1991b). *Training for Community Care. A Joint Approach*. London, HMSO.

SSI (1991c). *Hear Me: See Me. An Inspection of Services from Three Agencies to Disabled People in Gloucestershire*. London, DoH.

SSI (1992a). *Concern for Quality. The First Annual Report of the Chief Inspector, Social Services Inspectorate, 1991–92*. London, HMSO.

SSI (1992b). *Social Services for Hospital Patients I: Working at the Interface*. London, DoH.

SSI (1992c). *Social Services for Hospital Patients II: The Implications for Community Care*. London, DoH.

SSI (1992d). *Managing Training in Social Services. An Inspection of Arrangements in Three Local Authorities*. London, DoH.

SSI (1992e). *Promoting Women. Management Development and Training for Women in Social Services Departments*. London, DoH.

SSI (1993a). *Raising the Standard. The Second Annual Report of the Chief Inspector, Social Services Inspectorate, 1992–93*. London, HMSO.

SSI (1993b). *Whose Life Is It Anyway? A Report of an Inspection of Services for People with Multiple Impairments*. London, DoH.

SSI (1993c). *Social Services for Hospital Patients III: Users' and Carers' Perspective*. London, DoH.

SSI (1993d). *No Longer Afraid*. London, DoH.

SSI (1993e). *The Inspection of the Complaints Procedures in Local Authority Social Services Departments*. London, DoH.

Stanton, A. (1989). *Invitation to Self-management*. Ruislip, Dab Hand Press.

Staton, J. (1993). 'The gentle touch', *Community Care*, 9 December, 28–9.

Stevenson, O. (1989). 'Taken from home', in S. Shardlow (ed.) *The Values of Change in Social Work*. London, Tavistock.

Stevenson, O. and Parsloe, P. (1993). *Community Care and Empowerment*. York, Joseph Rowntree Foundation.

Stewart, I. (1991). 'Psychiatry: on its best behaviour', in P. Barker and S. Baldwin (eds) *Ethical Issues in Mental Health*. London, Chapman and Hall.

Stone, R. (1992). 'Mental Illness Specific Grant – new money?', *Openmind*, **57**, 5.

Stratton, P., Preston-Shoot, M. and Hanks, H. (1990). *Family Therapy Training and Practice*. Birmingham, Venture Press.

Stuart, O. (1993). 'Double oppression: an appropriate starting point?', in J. Swain, V. Finkelstein, S. French and M. Oliver (eds) *Disabling Barriers – Enabling Environments*. Milton Keynes, Open University/Sage.

Survivors Speak Out (1986). *We're Not Mad, We're Angry*. London, Channel 4 Television.

Sutherland, V. and Cooper, C. (1992). 'Job stress, satisfaction, and mental health among general practitioners before and after the introduction of new contract', *British Medical Journal*, **304**, 13 June, 1545–8.

Swain, J., Finkelstein, V., French, S. and Oliver, M. (1993). 'Introduction', in J. Swain, V. Finkelstein, S. French and M. Oliver (eds) *Disabling Barriers – Enabling Environments*. Milton Keynes, Open University/Sage.

Taylor, D. (1989). 'Citizenship and social power', *Critical Social Policy*, **26**, 9(2), 19–31.

Thompson, C. (1991). *Changing the Balance. Power and People Who Use Services*. London, NCVO.

Thompson, N. (1993). *Anti-Discriminatory Practice*. London, Macmillan.

Timms, N. (1983). *Social Work Values: an Enquiry*. London, RKP.

Timms, N. (1989). 'Social work values: context and contribution', in S. Shardlow (ed.) *The Values of Change in Social Work*. London, Tavistock.

Tunnard, J. (1991). 'Setting the scene for partnership', in Family Rights Group, *The Children Act 1989: Working in Partnership with Families*. Reader. London, HMSO.

UPIAS (1976). *Fundamental Principles of Disability*. London, UPIAS.

User Centred Services Group (1993). *Building Bridges between People Who Use and People Who Provide Services*. London, NISW.

Ussher, J. (1991). *Women's Madness. Misogyny or Mental Illness*. London, Harvester Wheatsheaf.

Values into Action (1992). *When the Eagles Fly*. London, VIA.

Values into Action (1993a). *The Resettlement Game*. London, VIA.

Values into Action (1993b). 'The easy life assessment guidelines', in S. Croft and P. Beresford (eds) *Getting Involved. A Practical Manual*. London, Open Services Project.

Victor, C. (1991). *Health and Health Care in Later Life*. Buckingham, Open University Press.

Wallcraft, J. (1993). 'Common issues and differences in user involvement across the country', in NHSTD, *Training and User Involvement in Mental Health Services*. London, National Health Service Training Directorate with Survivors Speak Out, Mindlink and National Advocacy Network.

Walmsley, J. (1993). '"Talking to top people": some issues relating to the citizenship of people with learning difficulties', in J. Swain, V. Finkelstein, S. French and M. Oliver (eds) *Disabling Barriers – Enabling Environments*. London, Open University/Sage.

Walmsley, J., Reynolds, J., Shakespeare, P. and Woolfe, R. (1993). 'Introduction', in J. Walmsley, J. Reynolds, P. Shakespeare and R. Woolfe (eds) *Health, Welfare and Practice. Reflecting on Roles and Relationships*. London, Sage/The Open University.

Warburton, R. (1990). *Developing Services for Disabled People. Results of an Inspection to Monitor the Operation of the Disabled Persons (Services, Consultation and Representation) Act 1986*. London, SSI/DoH.

Ward, D. and Mullender, A. (1991). 'Empowerment and oppression: an indissoluble pairing for contemporary social work', *Critical Social Policy*, **11**(2), 21–30.

Ward, L. (1991). 'Having a say in community care', *Community Care*, 11 April, 19.

Wardhaugh, J. and Wilding, P. (1993). 'Towards an explanation of the corruption of care', *Critical Social Policy*, 13(1), 4–31.

Webb-Johnson, A. (1991), *A Cry for Change. An Asian Perspective on Developing Quality Mental Health Care*. London, Conference of Indian Organisations.

Wertheimer, A. (1993). 'User participation in community care: the challenge for services', in V. Williamson (ed.) *Users first. The Real Challenge for Community Care*. Brighton, University of Brighton.

Westland, P. (1992). 'Decisions, decisions', *Community Care* (inside supplement), 27 February, v–vi.

Which? (1993). '*Which?* guide to NHS complaints', *Which?*, April, 14–15.

Whitfield, J. and Stewart, J. (1991). 'Service with a smile', *Community Care*, 19 September, 20–2.

Whitfield, J. and Stewart, J. (1993). 'Sound footings', *Community Care*, 'inside supplement, *Contracting*', 28 January, i–ii.

Whittington, C. (1971). 'Self-determination re-examined', *British Journal of Social Work*, **1**(3), 293–303.

Whittington, C. (1977). 'Social workers' orientations: an action perspective', *British Journal of Social Work*, **7**(1), 73–95.

Wiener, R. (1989). 'Stress within the team', *Social Work Today*, **20**(35), 20–1.

Wilding, P. (1982). *Professional Power and Social Welfare*. London, RKP.

Williams, J. (1991). 'Taking care of staff', in M. Marshall, M. Preston-Shoot and E. Wincott (eds) *Effective Management*. Birmingham, British Association of Social Workers.

Williams, J. (1993). 'What is a profession? Experience versus expertise', in J. Walmsley, J. Reynolds, P. Shakespeare and R. Woolfe (eds) *Health, Welfare and Practice. Reflecting on Roles and Relationships*. Milton Keynes, Open University/Sage.

Williams, K. (1991). *Community Care: a Training Needs Handbook*. London, LBTC Training for Care.

Williamson, V. (1993). 'Users first: from policy to practice', in V. Williamson (ed.) *Users First. The Real Challenge for Community Care*. Brighton, University of Brighton.

Wilson, D. (1992). *A Strategy of Change*. London, Routledge.

Winkler, F. (1990). 'Consumerism and information', in L. Winn (ed.) *Power to the People. The Key to Responsive Services in Health and Social Care*. London, The Kings Fund Centre.

Winn, L. and Chotai, N. (1990). 'Community development: working with black and ethnic minority groups', in L. Winn (ed.) *Power to the People. The Key to Responsive Services in Health and Social Care*. London, The Kings Fund Centre.

Wistow, G. (1993). 'Democratic deficit', *Community Care*, 30 September, 29.

Wistow, G. and Hardy, B. (1993). 'Managing the mixed economy of care', in D. Robbins (ed.) *Community Care. Findings from Department of Health Funded Research, 1988–1992*. London, HMSO.

Wistow, G., Hardy, B. and Leedham, I. (1993). 'Where do we go from here?', *Community Care*, 21 January, 20–1.

Witton, M. (1992). 'When variety is not working', *Community Care*, 3 December, 24–5.

Wolfensberger, W. (1972). *The Principle of Normalisation in Human Services*. Toronto, National Institute of Mental Retardation.

Wolfensberger, W. (1983). 'Social role valorisation: a proposed new term for the principle of normalisation', *Mental Retardation*, December, 234–9.

Women in Mind (1986). *Finding Our Own Solutions*. London, Mind.

Woolfe, R. (1992). 'Coping with stress', in T. Hobbs (ed.) *Experiential Training*. London, Routledge.

Author index

Subject index

COMMUNITY PROFILING
AUDITING SOCIAL NEEDS

Murray Hawtin, Geraint Hughes, Janie Percy-Smith with Anne Foreman

Social auditing and community profiles are increasingly being used in relation to a number of policy areas, including: housing, community care, community health, urban regeneration and local economic development. *Community Profiling* provides a practical guide to the community profiling process which can be used by professionals involved in the planning and delivery of services, community workers, community organizations, voluntary groups and tenants' associations. In addition it will provide an invaluable step-by-step guide to social science students involved in practical research projects.

The book takes the reader through the community profiling process beginning with consideration of what a community profile is, defining aims and objectives and planning the research. It then looks at a variety of methods for collecting, storing and analysing information and ways of involving the local community. Finally it considers how to present the information and develop appropriate action-plans. The book also includes a comprehensive annotated bibliography of recent community profiles and related literature.

Contents
What is a community profile? – Planning a community profile – Involving the community – Making use of existing information – Collecting new information – Survey methods – Storing and analysing data – Collating and presenting information – Not the end – Annotated bibliography – Index.

208pp   0 335 19113 4 (Paperback)

IMPLEMENTING COMMUNITY CARE

Nigel Malin (ed.)

This introductory text provides a unique overview of the implementation of community care policy and the process of managing changes in the field. The central thesis is an expansion of the theme of integrating policy and professional practice in order to assess the requirements for providing models of care based upon a user and care management perspective. The book analyses the impact of changes for community nurses, social workers, those employed in residential and home-based care and discusses anticipated new roles and functions. Its examination of changes in policy and planning both at national and local level makes it a valuable sourcebook for health care, social work practitioners and planners, but the volume is designed for use by students and professionals alike. The emphasis throughout is on the design and delivery of services and providing an overview of research findings, particularly in relation to measuring service effectiveness.

Contents
Preface – Section 1: The policy context – Development of community care – Management and finance – Community care planning – Care management – Section 2: Staff and users – The caring professions – The family and informal care – Measuring service quality – The consumer role – Section 3: Models of care – Residential services – Day services – Domiciliary services – Index.

Contributors
Andy Alaszewski, Michael Beazley, John Brown, David Challis, Brian Hardy, Bob Hudson, Aileen McIntosh, Steve McNally, Nigel Malin, Jill Manthorpe, Jim Monarch, John Rose, Len Spriggs, Gerald Wistow, Wai-Ling Wun.

224pp   0 335 15738 6 (Paperback)   0 335 15739 4 (Hardback)

EVALUATING COMMUNITY CARE
SERVICES FOR PEOPLE WITH LEARNING DIFFICULTIES

Ken Wright, Alan Haycox and Ian Leedham

The aim of this book is to describe and discuss the principles of evaluating community care services for people with learning difficulties and to explore how they have been applied in the development of policy in the last ten years. Although the contents are based heavily upon the theory and practice of micro-economic appraisal of health and social care, other social science disciplines are exploited wherever relevant. No prior knowledge of any of these disciplines is expected. The coverage of the book follows the logical steps in policy evaluation including an explanation of different approaches to evaluation, a discussion of recent policy objectives, the measurement of outcomes and costs and the policy implications of recent evaluative studies. The book concludes with an examination of the relevance of evaluative studies to the new arrangements for community care of people with learning difficulties.

Contents
Introduction – The evaluation framework – The policy background – Outcomes 1: definition and methodology – Outcomes 2: specific research dimensions and their measurement – Outcomes 3: evidence and issues – Cost measurement in theory – Cost measurement in practice – Conclusion: policy development and evaluation in the 1990s – References – Index.

208pp   0 335 09496 1 (Paperback)   0 335 09497 X (Hardback)